D1354246

0 0 0 0 0 5 3 2

KEYBOARD, GRAPHIC AND HANDWRITING SKILLS

FORTHCOMING TITLES

Occupational Therapy for the Brain-Injured Adult
Jo Clark-Wilson and Gordon Muir Giles

Multiple Sclerosis
Approaches to management
Lorraine De Souza

Modern Electrotherapy
Mary Dyson and Christopher Hayne

Physiotherapy in Respiratory and Intensive Care
Alexandra Hough

Understanding Dysphasia
Lesley Jordan and Rita Twiston Davies

Management in Occupational Therapy
Zielfa B. Maslin

Dysarthria
Theory and therapy
Sandra J. Robertson

Speech and Language Problems in Children
Dilys A. Treharne

Occupational Therapy in Rheumatology
Lynne Sandles

Limb Amputation
From aetiology to rehabilitation
Rosalind Ham and Leonard Cotton

THERAPY IN PRACTICE SERIES
Edited by Jo Campling

This series of books is aimed at 'therapists' concerned with rehabilitation in a very broad sense. The intended audience particularly includes occupational therapists, physiotherapists and speech therapists, but many titles will also be of interest to nurses, psychologists, medical staff, social workers, teachers or volunteer workers. Some volumes are interdisciplinary, others are aimed at one particular profession. All titles will be comprehensive but concise, and practical but with due reference to relevant theory and evidence. They are not research monographs but focus on professional practice, and will be of value to both students and qualified personnel.

1. Occupational Therapy for Children with Disabilities
   Dorothy E. Penso
2. Living Skills for Mentally Handicapped People
   Christine Peck and Chia Swee Hong
3. Rehabilitation of the Older Patient
   Edited by Amanda J. Squires
4. Physiotherapy and the Elderly Patient
   Paul Wagstaff and Davis Coakley
5. Rehabilitation of the Severely Brain-Injured Adult
   Edited by Ian Fussey and Gordon Muir Giles
6. Communication Problems in Elderly People
   Rosemary Gravell
7. Occupational Therapy Practice in Psychiatry
   Linda Finlay
8. Working with Bilingual Language Disability
   Edited by Deirdre M. Duncan
9. Counselling Skills for Health Professionals
   Philip Burnard
10. Teaching Interpersonal Skills
    A handbook of experiential learning for health professionals
    Philip Burnard
11. Occupational Therapy for Stroke Rehabilitation
    Simon Thompson and Maryanne Morgan
12. Assessing Physically Disabled People at Home
    Kathy Maczka
13. Acute Head Injury
    Practical management in rehabilitation
    Ruth Garner
14. Practical Physiotherapy with Older People
    Lucinda Smyth et al.
15. Keyboard, Graphic and Handwriting Skills
    Helping people with motor disabilities
    Dorothy E. Penso
16. Community Occupational Therapy with Mentally Handicapped Adults
    Debbie Isaac
17. Autism
    Professional perspectives and practice
    Edited by Kathryn Ellis

Keyboard, Graphic and Handwriting Skills

Helping people with motor disabilities

Senior Occupational Therapist,
Child Development Centre,
York District Hospital, UK

CHAPMAN AND HALL
London • New York • Tokyo • Melbourne • Madras

UK	Chapman and Hall, 11 New Fetter Lane, London EC4P 4EE
USA	Chapman and Hall, 29 West 35th Street, New York NY10001
Japan	Chapman and Hall Japan, Thomson Publishing Japan, Hirakawacho Nemoto Building, 7F, 1-7-11 Hirakawa-cho, Chiyoda-ku, Tokyo 102
Australia	Chapman and Hall Australia, Thomas Nelson Australia, 480 La Trobe Street, PO Box 4725, Melbourne 3000
India	Chapman and Hall India, R. Sheshadri, 32 Second Main Road, CIT East, Madras 600 035

First edition 1990

© 1990 Dorothy E. Penso

Typeset in 10/12pt Times by Mayhew Typesetting, Bristol
Printed in Great Britain by St Edmundsbury Press Ltd,
Bury St Edmunds, Suffolk

ISBN 0 412 32210 2

British Library Cataloguing in Publication Data
Penso, Dorothy E.
  Keyboard graphic and handwriting skills: helping people with
  motor disabilities. — (Therapy in practice)
1. Motor disordered persons, rehabilitation
  I. Title II. Series
  362.1'967

  ISBN 0 412 32210 2

Library of Congress Cataloging-in-Publication Data
Penso, Dorothy E., 1837–
  Keyboard, graphic, and handwriting skills : helping people with motor
disabilities / Dorothy E. Penso.
     p. cm. — (Therapy in practice series : 15)
  Includes bibliographical references.
  ISBN 0 412 32210 2 (pbk.)
    1. Movement disorders — Patients — Rehabilitation. 2. Movement
disorders in children — Patients — Rehabilitation. 3. Occupational
therapy. 4. Motor ability. 5. Penmanship. 6. Electronic data processing
— Keyboarding. I. Title. II. Series.
    [DNLM: 1. Art. 2. Handwriting. 3. Motor Skills. 4. Movement
Disorders — rehabilitation. 5. Word Processing. WL 390 P418k]
  RC376.5.P46   1990
  616.7'3 — dc20
  DNLM/DLC   89-70845
  for Library of Congress   CIP

Contents

Acknowledgements   ix

Foreword   xi

1 Introduction: what people wish to record on paper and the disabilities which impair their ability to do so   1

2 First steps towards handwriting, graphic and keyboard skills   11

3 Assessment: defining needs and problems   23

4 Positioning: people and work surfaces   46

5 Pens, pencils and brushes   60

6 Tools and techniques for artwork   73

7 Typewriters and electronic printers: teaching keyboard skills   95

8 Microcomputers for word processing and graphics   126

References   148

Further reading   151

Appendix A: Glossary of microcomputing terms   155

Appendix B: Glossary of medical terms   158

Appendix C: Suppliers   161

Index   166

Acknowledgements

During my career as an occupational therapist I have exchanged ideas and discussed problems with many colleagues. Many of my clients and their families have discussed their difficulties with me and tested my ideas for helping them to overcome them. Many have solved their own problems and have passed on their ingenious solutions to me. I thank all these people for sharing their experiences, ideas and opinions with me.

A number of people have given me permission to reproduce their drawings, handwriting and keyboard work. I thank them for allowing me to share their difficulties, and sometimes the solutions to these difficulties, with others.

I would like to thank Terry Winston who interpreted my ideas and drew many of the illustrations. My thanks to Nottingham Rehab and, in particular, to Mr L.C. Graham for the loan of equipment for evaluation and permission to reproduce illustrations from their catalogue as line drawings. Mr Clive Jenkins of Jenx Limited answered numerous questions about the Jenx Prone Angle Chair and kindly provided a line drawing of it.

Malcolm Brunton, of the Medical Physics Department, York District Hospital, has patiently helped me to become proficient with the use of microcomputers, in particular with word processing, and has always been ready to find solutions to both my own difficulties with microcomputers and those of my clients.

I am grateful to Jo Campling, series editor, and Christine Birdsall, editor, for their support and encouragement during the preparation of this book.

Foreword

The practising paediatrician struggles to combat the effects of acute illness and disease in babies and older children. The pattern of hospital admissions has changed dramatically since I first qualified over 25 years ago. Neonatology is a relatively new branch of paediatrics and achievements in neonatal intensive care have been exciting and little short of astonishing. However, like the poor, children with chronic disabilities are always with us. Sadly, modern mainstream medical progressive thinkers regard as much less prestigious the work done in the field of 'handicap'.

Thanks to inspirational paediatricians, like Ronnie McKeith, Trevor Wright and Ray Remboldt (great teachers all, and wise counsellors to learners like myself), the needs of children with developmental disabilities have been highlighted. Moreover, the importance of a holistic approach to these children, their families and their teachers has been emphasized.

In the Child Development Centre at York, a multidisciplinary team attempts to define as accurately as possible the nature and severity of the problems facing a child, but the child's predicament and how to solve or alleviate it remains the key issue. A full team assessment which does not lead to any practical help for the child and his family is merely an academic exercise and a disgrace to the many different professions involved.

Each child is unique and no management blueprint is at hand after each assessment. In her first book *Occupational Therapy for Children with Disabilities*, Dorothy Penso not only outlined the extent and range of developmental problems facing the children whom she meets in her daily work, but also discussed assessment and treatment plans.

In this, her second book, *Keyboard, Graphic and Handwriting Skills: Helping people with motor disabilities* she narrows the field and sharpens the focus. Theories on learning disabilities are always interesting to the specialist with an enquiring mind and her Further Reading section will undoubtedly appeal to workers in this field. However, the practical basis of this book will, I feel, be its principal attraction and its enduring value.

I welcome those advances which enable children and adults with disabilities to make the sort of progress they and their families scarcely dreamed possible ten short years ago and I am grateful to all those children, parents, therapists and teachers who have opened my blinkered eyes to a computerized world that I do not myself comprehend.

Our rich section of the world worships ever more the big, the wealthy and the so-called intelligent. Man can go to the moon, yet the malformed, the retarded and the disabled can be considered disposable by so many of our fellow citizens.

When staff from the disparate fields of health, education and social services share ideas, much can be done to redress this imbalance. Dorothy Penso herself was the beneficiary of a Regional Hospital Authority research grant which enabled her to study at first hand work carried out in Child Development Centers in the USA.

Child Development Centre patients benefit greatly from the efforts of conscientious enthusiasts and amazingly generous voluntary bodies. Much remains to be done.

Dorothy Penso's second book is another step on the road to the abolition of prejudice against the handicapped child. I thank her for all she has taught me and I wish this book well. Dorothy has been a tireless advocate of the rights of disabled children and their families and I salute her for this. She fulfils as an excellent occupational therapist the aims of the Good Physician, 'To cure – but seldom, to alleviate – often, to comfort – always'.

Hugh J. Heggarty MB ChB FRCP
Consultant Paediatrician

1

Introduction: what people wish to record on paper and the disabilities which impair their ability to do so

Men trust their ears less than their eyes
Herodotus, 5th century BC

Paintings on the walls of caves inhabited by people thousands of years ago (Blakemore, 1988), illuminated manuscripts preserved from the Middle Ages, declarations of love carved on Victorian lace bobbins, the first attempts of four-year-old children to write their names; for thousands of years people have had a strong desire to make their mark, more or less permanently, on paper and other materials.

People wish to record both graphics and words. Some record only the small amounts necessary in day-to-day life, recording words or diagrams for personal use or to communicate with others. Some people need to record in the course of paid employment, others because of an overwhelming desire to communicate with other people, perhaps even aiming for publication.

The ease with which this recording is accomplished varies, and depends on many skills including motor ability. A large proportion of the population has no physical impediment to its recording skills. The remainder has a greater or lesser degree of impairment which impedes or prevents recording on paper. Some people are limited in the modes of recording which they may employ and require adapted writing and drawing tools or even sophisticated electronic devices.

Were it not for such devices and the resourcefulness of the author, his family, teachers and peers, we would not be able to read today Christopher Nolan's *Dam-burst of Dreams* and *Under the Eye of the Clock* (Nolan, 1981, 1987). The latter provides a magnificent insight into the nature of the disabilities caused by severe cerebral palsy, which is more explicit than many medical textbooks. When the amount of effort which is required for Christopher Nolan to record just one word is considered, it will be appreciated just how strong his desire to record his thoughts and memories must be.

Consider also Joseph Deacon who, after the death of his mother during his childhood, lived the remainder of his life in a hospital for those with mental handicap and because of his motor disability and expressive language difficulty never received formal education. Despite these obstacles, during his adult life he wrote his autobiography with the help of three fellow patients, one who could understand his dysarthric speech and who passed his words on to a second who could spell and in turn passed the spelling of his words to a third who could type but not spell (Deacon, 1974). Such is the strength of desire experienced by some people to record on paper, that they will seek to overcome severe disability in order to do so. Not all have such severe disability, yet there are many children and adults who benefit from the careful selection of appropriate tools and equipment to enable the development and furthering of recording skills. Understanding the usual sequence of events in the development of recording skills will aid the choice of equipment and skills for those who have impairments which impede recording on paper.

An infant of 15 months provided with an appropriate tool will mark a surface in imitation of an adult's pencil strokes. The young child will delight in applying colour to paper. Adults may enquire of the child as to what the colours represent. In fact it is not anything but pleasure in marking paper in a unique fashion, the joy of practising manual skill, coordination of hand and eye, and choice in colour and shape.

First attempts at representation on paper may be recognizable only to the originator. The skill of motor planning, of directing the hand accurately have not yet been learned nor have the devices used to represent space and distance, relative size and perspective. These skills will develop to a greater or lesser degree as the child matures.

By the time most children are of school age they have the necessary motor and perceptual skills to begin to copy the system of symbols, letter characters, which is used to record and communicate on paper and other materials. At first the child concentrates on the production of recognizable letter characters; their formation requires conscious motor planning (praxis). By the age of eight, children are usually able to give all their attention to the content of their written work, the mechanics of writing having been learned, the accurate formation of letter characters and words requires no conscious effort. They, of course, differ in the degree of enthusiasm with which they undertake writing and drawing tasks. Most children who are provided with suitable materials will enjoy experimenting with colour and shape; they will make representations of people and objects, situations and events.

Children of school age are required to use recording skills of increasing complexity as their education progresses. They will be required to record on paper in the following ways:

1. Copying written information from chalkboards and books.
2. Writing matter which is dictated to them.
3. Composing pieces of imaginative writing.
4. Extracting the essence of what is said to them by their teachers, has been viewed on television or observed in a laboratory and recording it in note form on paper.
5. Writing legibly and at speed in examinations. (Examinations written at a 15 and 16 year old level require a writing speed of between 16 and 20 words per minute if an adequate amount of information is to be recorded (Chasty, 1986).)
6. Setting out mathematical problems logically in words and numbers.
7. Drawing graphs, maps and diagrams and labelling them appropriately.
8. Tracing maps and pictures.
9. Colouring in outline pictures.
10. Using rulers, set squares, protractors and compasses.
11. Composing pictures and patterns using pencils, crayons, pens, inks, and various types of paint.

The years of formal eduction are, for most people, the time of greatest output of material recorded on paper. Today, fewer people are employed in occupations which require them, for most of the day, to write or produce designs on paper by means of a pen or pencil. The days are gone when firms employed teams of clerks and bookkeepers who wrote in ledgers and day books. Today, increasing use is being made of microcomputers and other devices. They are used by engineers, draughtsmen and other designers. In shops the price tags are printed, not inscribed by hand. The telephone is used to a larger extent than in the past; many people make telephone calls rather than communicate by letter. Library catalogues are no longer laboriously handwritten on index cards but recorded on microfiche.

Despite this radical change in the working life of many people, there are still many occasions when it is necessary for adults to be able to record on paper. Indeed, life is fraught with frustrations and embarrassments for people who are unable to do so. People will go to endless trouble to conceal the fact that they have difficulty with handwriting. Handwriting is by no means an obsolete skill.

What are the recording skills employed by adults?

1. Adults often need to sign their names on cheques, receipts, pension and benefit books. Not only is there dignity in being able to sign ones name, but in many instances the ability to do so enables personal and financial transactions to be undertaken privately.
2. People write shopping lists, leave written messages for other people, make notes on calendars and in diaries, note addresses and telephone numbers, write greetings cards etc.
3. Letters are written which are private to the sender and recipient.
4. Many employers prefer job application forms to be filled in by hand rather than with a typewriter.
5. Most people are required to complete income tax returns and other official forms. These, of course, may be completed with the help of a typewriter though it is quite a skilled task aligning the type characters in the small spaces provided for responses to questions.
6. There is an increasing number of people who are interested in creative writing as a hobby or as a profession. People write factual articles, short stories, novels and poems.
7. There are those who create pictures with pen, pencil, water or oil paints, pastels, crayons and other media for their own pleasure and also as a profession.
8. People wish to draw technical diagrams and decorative graphics, both for domestic use and as a profession.

There are a number of both children and adults who find some or all tasks which involve recording on paper more than usually difficult, and in some cases impossible to accomplish and could be helped by the selection of suitable tools or the provision of a typewriter or microcomputer. The people who experience these difficulties may be divided into two groups.

1. Those who have never had the ability to record on paper because of disability which was congenital or occurred early in life.
2. Those who have had normal ability to record on paper but because of trauma or disease have lost that ability.

CONGENITAL DISABILITY, DISABILITY ACQUIRED IN THE FIRST YEARS OF LIFE

The outlook for children with serious congenital disability is considerably brighter than it was in the past, because both the nature of their disability and their potential is appreciated to a greater extent today. The likelihood of difficulty with recording on paper is usually anticipated, fewer children with disabilities continue for years the often futile struggle to manipulate pens and pencils effectively (O'Hare and Brown, 1989). Measures are taken to find alternative methods of recording, such as electric and electronic typewriters, microcomputers with a word processing facility, visual display and appropriate controls. This technology has enabled many children to demonstrate their ability to assimilate knowledge, their understanding of concepts and their creative potential.

There are, however, adults who have spent all or most of their lives suffering from disability who, when young, did not have the advantages that children have today. Such people have had little opportunity, until recent years, to develop the skills necessary to be able to record on paper.

There are many types of congenital disability which inhibit recording on paper.

1. Complete or partial deficiency of upper limbs.
2. Disturbance of the control of movement which occurs in conditions such as cerebral palsy and may be manifested as spasticity, athetosis or ataxia. The severity of these conditions varies between sufferers. Some may need only minor adaptations to tools and equipment, whilst others will need custom-made electronic devices to allow recording on paper to take place.
3. Hemiplegia is of particular significance if it occurs in what would have been the innately preferred hand for, obviously, that hand cannot be used for writing and other fine motor skills. The affected person will be using the non-preferred hand for fine motor tasks. This possibility should always be considered when assessing the hand skills of people suffering from congenital hemiplegia. It is frequently found that fine hand skills on the unaffected side are poor when compared with those of the average person. This may be the result of the hand not affected by hemiplegia being used as the preferred hand which would not have been so had there been no neurological deficit on the other side of the body. Alternatively, it may be that the dysfunction

5

Figure 1.1: Samples of the handwriting of a girl who suffers from arthrogryposis and non-progressive muscle atrophy. a) At 6.5 years and b) at 8.5 years. Her inter-phalangeal joints may be passively but not actively flexed. She holds her pen in her right hand in the cleft between her extended index and middle fingers. The speed of her writing is normal for her chronological age. Note the slight unsteadiness in her writing.

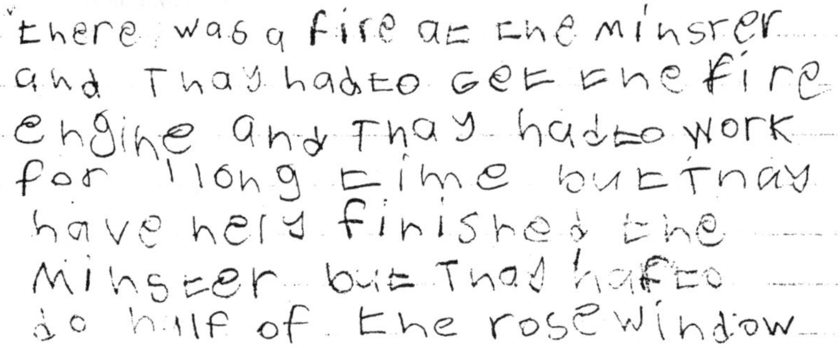

there was a fire at the minster
and Thay hadto get the fire
engine and Thay hadto work
for llong time but Tnay
have herd finished the
Minster but Thad hafto
do half of the rose window

(a)

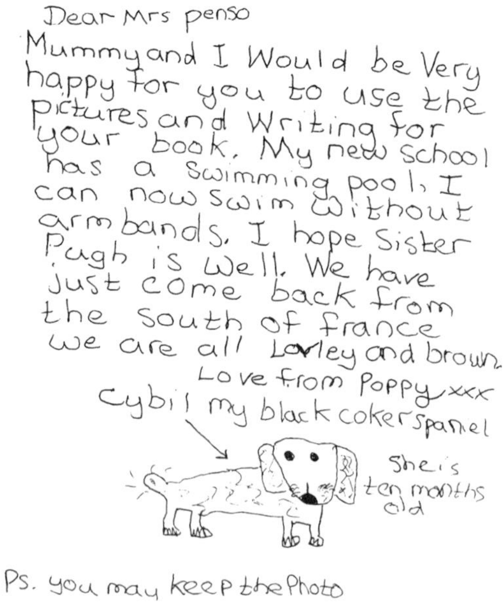

Dear Mrs penso
Mummy and I would be very
happy for you to use the
pictures and writing for
your book. My new school
has a swimming pool, I
can now swim without
arm bands. I hope sister
Pugh is well. We have
just come back from
the south of france
we are all lovley and brown.
Love from Poppy xxx
Cybil my black coker spaniel
She is ten months old

Ps. you may keep the Photo

(b)

which prevents the innately preferred hand being used also affects the other hand to some lesser degree.

4. Dystonia has been described as 'a syndrome of sustained muscle contractions, frequently causing twisting and repetitive movements, or abnormal postures' (Herxheimer, 1988). Only the briefest handwriting is usually possible and adaptations may be necessary if a keyboard is to be used effectively. Symptoms are sometimes exacerbated when the sufferer is being observed.

5. Poor muscle power which occurs in the muscular atrophies and dystrophies makes handwriting arduous. Many of these conditions are progressive and provision of alternative methods of recording should be made before handwriting skills are completely lost and the alternative means becomes essential.

6. Limitation of movement which occurs in diseases such as arthrogryposis, a connective tissue disorder and osteogenesis imperfecta (brittle bones). Many people who suffer from such conditions devise their own unique method of controlling a pen or pencil (Figure 1.1). Where large amounts of written work are necessary a keyboard is usually the best tool to use. A mini-keyboard is helpful where range of movement is limited.

7. Dyspraxia, difficulty with planning movements despite normal muscle power, sensation and comprehension of the task to be performed. It may occur in isolation or as a symptom of cerebral palsy, spina bifida or specific learning difficulties. Sufferers may have great difficulty with the movements required for hand-writing, they will have difficulty learning from completed examples of letter characters and words. Such people may need to have the movements necessary to form letter characters demonstrated many times, preferably with a verbal commentary, before they are able to learn them. Where large amounts of writing are required a keyboard which removes the need for precise and varied motor planning is often the most successful means of recording on paper.

ACQUIRED DISABILITY

There are also people who have spent part of their life enjoying normal motor ability and have had no difficulty with fine motor skills. At some point in their life, trauma or disease has impaired fine motor and other skills making writing, drawing and other fine hand skills difficult or impossible to accomplish. There are many types of acquired disability which impair the ability to record on paper.

1. Loss of part or all of the preferred hand. People differ in the amount of difficulty they experience in acquiring handwriting and drawing skills in the non-preferred hand. A keyboard, using special fingering for one hand, may become the most realistic method of recording for all but the briefest of notes and signatures.

2. Pain and limitation of hand movement due to conditions such as arthritis. Adapted pens and pencils which reduce joint strain and allow adequate grip where joint movement is limited may be helpful for brief writing tasks. A keyboard may be the most realistic solution for the person who must complete large amounts of written work. A good overall position is especially important when a keyboard is used for prolonged periods so that unnecessary joint strain does not occur. A keyguard or a forearm support will also help to prevent strain on the joints of the wrist and hand.

3. Loss of muscle power occurs in conditions such as muscular atrophy and muscular dystrophy which present during adolescence and early adult life. Writing tools, such as soft felt-tipped pens, which readily mark the paper with the need to exert only minimal pressure, may be helpful. Often a keyboard is the best method of recording on paper and, as with the types of muscular dystrophy which present earlier in life, it is best to learn keyboard skills while handwriting is still a useful skill rather than wait until a keyboard becomes the only method by which the sufferer can record on paper.

4. Tremor, which occurs in diseases such as multiple sclerosis and Parkinson's disease, will make handwriting difficult to execute and difficult to read because of the tremor which will be apparent in the completed writing, unevenness and often the smallness of the writing (Figure 1.2). A keyboard with a keyguard will probably be the most effective means of recording on paper.

5. Cerebrovascular accident (CVA) resulting in spasticity or flaccidity of the preferred arm and hand. Some people may successfully establish handwriting in what has been the non-preferred hand. Others will find a keyboard a more appropriate means of recording on paper. People who have suffered CVA often suffer from verbal language impairment which may also affect their ability to record words and construct sentences on

Figure 1.2: The handwriting of an eighty year old man who suffers from Parkinsonism. a) Writing with a ball point pen. b) Writing with fibre tip pen. c) Writing with a Biocurve pen. He had kept a diary since childhood until recently when his hand became too unsteady for writing more than a few words. His preference was for the felt-tipped pen. He felt that the slightly thicker and heavier barrel helped hand stability. It would be interesting to see his handwriting using a Biocurve pen (Figure 5.7) which had a fibre tip which would provide more friction than the ball point which is presently available.

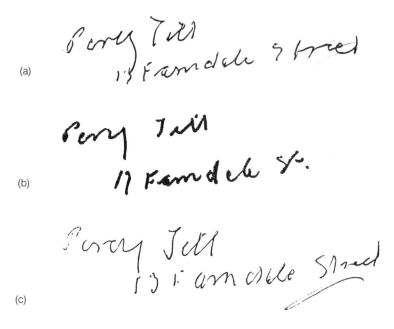

(a)

(b)

(c)

paper, others suffer perceptual impairment which is likely to affect recording skills.

Only a small number of disabling conditions are described above, but no matter what the condition which impairs a persons ability to record on paper, not only must the condition of the hands be taken into consideration; the whole body can also influence these abilities. Consider the difference in the quality of handwriting when any person writes whilst sitting back in an easy chair or resting the paper against a wall with that of the person when sitting at a table of suitable height with an appropriate chair. Differences will be seen in the quality of handwriting of the ablest person. Many disabling conditions make a conventional sitting position difficult or impossible. People who

9

suffer from conditions such as severe cerebral palsy, osteogenesis imperfecta or spina bifida not only have hand problems to contend with but also the general positioning of the body and the co-ordination of hand and eye.

Whether the problem is congenital or acquired, short term, continuing or degenerative, if means are to be devised which allow people with motor disabilities to record on paper effectively, it is essential to make a careful evaluation of their strengths and weaknesses and acquire an appreciation of the type of activity they wish to undertake, knowledge of the writing and drawing devices, types of keyboards and electronic devices which are available.

The following chapters will describe the development of abilities which are desirable when recording on paper, the assessment of those abilities, and some of the equipment and devices which may help those with motor disabilities to achieve their potential. It is not intended to discuss the teaching of handwriting, graphics or creative writing *per se*, but to suggest strategies and devices to help those people who have motor disabilities to record on paper what is required of them in the course of their daily life during educational, professional, domestic and leisure pursuits.

2

First steps towards handwriting, graphic and keyboard skills

The mighty hand leads to a sloping shoulder,
The finger joints are cramped with chalk;
Dylan Thomas

Recording on paper; drawing and other forms of design, handwriting, graphics, words produced by means of a keyboard, all require a variety of skills. Motor activity, at both a gross and fine level, is common to all these activities.

Recording on paper usually requires some degree of hand function. Exceptions are people unable to use their hands who learn to manipulate painting, writing or drawing tools with the feet, mouth or other part of the body. Other people who cannot describe the precise movements required for writing and graphic work, learn to operate an electric or electronic keyboard using various parts of the body or by sophisticated scanning or coding systems (Workman, Geggie and Creasey, 1988). Before conventional or exceptional input methods can be used, detailed assessment of the abilities of the individual concerned, together with evaluation of the equipment, is necessary.

This chapter considers the skills which are desirable in children and adults who hope to be able to use writing and drawing tools, keyboards and microcomputers to record on paper. Hand function is only one of many desirable skills; the stability of the whole of the body is involved, for the hand is of little use unless it has stability and is coordinated with the eyes.

GROSS MOTOR SKILLS

In order to coordinate hand and eye in all but a supine position, the position of the head must be controlled while the body is in a sitting or standing position. This head control is usually established by the age of 20 weeks (Illingworth, 1983; Sheridan, 1975). Control of the position of the head in relation to the trunk and limbs (righting reactions) becomes possible no matter what the position of the body. 'The function of righting reactions is the maintenance of the normal position of the head in space and the proper alignment of the head and neck with the trunk, and of the trunk with the limbs' (Bobath, 1974). Righting reactions usually begin to develop during the sixth month.

A controlled head position enables the eyes to coordinate with whatever task the hands are undertaking. True hand/eye coordination enables the eyes to monitor the task the hands are accomplishing; it does not mean that the eyes are monitoring the hands. For example when the average person is writing with a pen the eyes are monitoring what is being written, not the movements the hand and fingers are making in order to produce that writing. 'The eye follows the hand, checking its path, its formation and organises the direction and space beyond. The eye checks the limits of the writing space and ensures the correctness of the letter and word formations' (Burr, 1980).

For there to be good hand/eye coordination there must also be adequate perception of self, body image and spatial concepts resulting from the integration of sensory input and motor planning ability (pp. 25–6 and 30–31).

Usually, recording activities are undertaken whilst in a sitting or standing position. Independent sitting is usually accomplished by the age of 9 months and standing by about one year (Illingworth, 1983; Sheridan, 1975). This trunk stability, which is manifested by the ability to sit and stand independently, is also important if the arm is to be used effectively in its role of enabling hand function. A stable shoulder girdle provides a base for effective arm movement and its position also dictates the position of the upper arm. 'Without a stable trunk, the arm–hand unit cannot offer its best function' (Ayres, 1974).

For handwriting and drawing the hand is usually held in a position of approximately 45° supination, the exact degree of supination varying with the age of the subject. Ziviani, in her investigation into children's prehension while writing, suggests that 'the transition from print to cursive writing makes a slightly more supinated posture of the forearm advantageous' (Ziviani, 1982). The arm must be supported and directed by a stable shoulder girdle.

When operating a keyboard the hands are usually held in a pronated position with the wrists in slight extension. The reader may like to experiment using a keyboard with the wrists in various positions. It will be found that if the wrists are flexed instead of extended a greater degree of elbow flexion is required and that after a short while repeated finger movement with the wrists flexed becomes quite uncomfortable and stressful. This illustrates the importance of a good working position which facilitates an appropriate sitting or standing position with the work surface at a suitable height to allow this comfortable degree of wrist extension.

A slight degree of wrist extension is also employed when handwriting, the exact degree will be influenced by the angle of the surface on which the hand rests, the greatest wrist extension being evident when writing on a vertical surface. The exception to this slightly extended wrist posture is those who use a hooked hand, in which the wrist is flexed and results in the hand being held above the line of writing and the arm having a greater degree of abduction than when the hand holding the pen is held below the line of writing.

This hooked hand style of writing has been associated with left-handedness. The rationale being that the left-handed writer adopts this position so as to have a better view of what is being written. However, people who write with their right hands have also been observed to adopt this position. It has been suggested that 'writing position was related to cerebral dominance and indicated that the inverted position' (hooked hand) 'of left handed writers was associated with an ipsilateral language hemisphere and the non-inverted position with a contralateral language hemisphere' (Levy and Reid, 1976).

More recent research considers inverted hand posture as a strategy representing 'an adaptation to the necessity of writing with an adduction movement' (in left-handed writers) 'rather than the symptom of any neurological particularity' (Guiard and Millerat, 1984). Along with inverted hand posture other strategies are described: anti-clockwise rotation of the paper, horizontal orientation of the forearm of the writing hand and positioning of the non-writing hand just below the beginning of the line of writing.

Particularly when neurological impairment is involved, the reasons for left-handedness must be considered. Is the subject innately left-handed, has the left become the writing hand because of acquired impairment to the right hand, has the left hand always been used for fine motor tasks because it has better function than the right hand though the latter may be the innately preferred hand? Consideration should also be given to the observation that some people who choose to write with the right hand also adopt a hooked hand posture. It cannot be concluded that they do this in order to see more easily the current line of writing or that they are compensating for the adduction movement necessary for left-handed writers. The following case illustrates the experience of one neurologically impaired child who appears to be influenced by neurological patterning to adopt a right inverted hand posture whilst writing.

Nicholas, who suffers from cerebral palsy was, at the age of 7 years, having great difficulty mastering handwriting. His sharp sense of humour suggested that he was far more intelligent than he was able to illustrate on paper. At nursery school he had enjoyed the freedom of painting with a large brush though these early attempts lacked form and variety. Each day he presented his mother with a brown picture which be described as 'a cow's bed'. One day he presented her with a bright red picture. His mother anticipated a fresh subject. 'What have you painted today?' she asked. Nicholas replied, 'It's a fire - it's a cow's bed on fire!'

Nicholas was not able to display such wit in writing. He wrote laboriously with an acutely hooked right hand, forming letter characters from bottom to top. This posture had not been evident when he painted using a whole arm movement. His occupational therapist felt that this was unacceptable and would create great problems when he began to learn cursive script. Attempts were made to encourage a more conventional, slightly extended wrist position without success. A small wrist splint was made which held his wrist in the desired position. It was interesting that when his wrist was held in this position he adjusted his body and arm position so that he was still writing with his hand above the line of writing.

His handwriting continued to be slow and laborious. It was decided that a portable electronic typewriter would be a more suitable way for him to record on paper. Nicholas was quick to learn the keyboard and today, at the age of 10, can type more quickly than his peers are able to write and he is able to demonstrate his ability much more effectively on paper. As a result of learning to use a keyboard the slight behaviour problems which had been apparent in school, no doubt because of his frustration with his poor handwriting skills, have completely disappeared (Figure 2.1).

FINE MOTOR SKILLS

In the first weeks of life the fingers are held mainly in a flexed position. By three months the hand is held in a more open position and an object placed in it will be retained for a few seconds. A child of six months will voluntarily grasp a toy with a crude whole hand and fingers grip with the hand in a pronated position. Grip has not yet developed suitably for the manipulation of a writing or drawing tool, yet there are children and adults who are able only to use this type of whole hand grasp. It is possible to manipulate an adapted writing tool with this grip, either by adding a T-bar to the tool or by greatly enlarging the part which is gripped (Chapter 5).

By the time the child is ten months old the index finger will be used to poke at small objects and lead when reaching for or pointing at them. The child is beginning to isolate and use a single finger. At this time the child will involve both hands in the exploration of objects, passing them from one hand to the other. The child is involved in two handed activity which is desirable for handwriting, drawing and keyboard skills. At about 15 months this extended index finger will be used in apposition with the thumb to pick up small objects. The child has the beginnings of the grip required to hold and manipulate a writing or drawing tool. Yet when the child first attempts to mark paper it will be with the tool held in a fisted hand.

Hand function required to manipulate a pen, pencil or brush efficiently

Provided with adequate opportunity, a child of 15 months will hold a crayon with a whole hand ulnar grip and mark a piece of paper with it in imitation of a mark demonstrated by another person and sometimes even spontaneously. The movement will not be isolated to the fingers or even the hand but will be a whole arm movement.

By the age of approximately two and a half years the grip will have moved from the ulnar to the radial side of the hand with the index finger extending down the barrel of the tool. There will still be arm movement involved in the manipulation of the tool. It is not until the average child is about seven years old that the pen is manipulated by means of a dynamic tripod grip (Ziviani, 1982). This means the manipulation of the tool will be accomplished by movement of the fingers alone. It is with this type of grip that the tool will be used effectively to describe letter characters evenly and swiftly.

Recording on paper is not a static task and requires more than efficient grip of the tool. The underlying ability required is that of moving the tool over the paper in a variety of directions to achieve the desired effects, pictorial representations or letter characters.

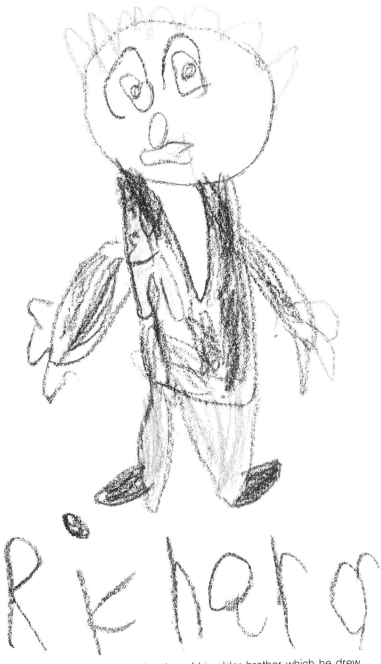

Figure 2.1: a) Nicholas's drawing of his elder brother which he drew one week before his fifth birthday. The content of the drawing is very mature for his chronological age, including details like eye pupils and brows, two dimensional limbs and facial features, though his difficulty with fine motor control is apparent.

At the lake district there or is a lot of hills.

Nicholas Dobson Nicholas Dobson

b) Nicholas's handwriting at eight years of age which he produced very slowly with a great deal of effort. It was obviously not an appropriate method for him to use for recording on paper.

```
Nicholas Dobson

For the weekend I am going to London

to visit my Auntie Irene and uncle

Charles and Brutus.

We will be playing football on the

beach sometimes and sometimes we wont.
```

c) An example of a small piece of Nicholas's typewriting which he produced quickly and easily when he was nine years old. He will need to use a small easily portable electric typewriter when he moves to secondary school and needs to move to a different classroom for each lesson.

There are conditions where this variety of movement is impaired by lack of power, limitation of joint movement, tremor, fluctuating muscle tone, pain or dyspraxia. Careful assessment of abilities and discussion with the person concerned will enable decisions to be made about the type and amount of recording desired and the appropriateness of the various methods of recording on paper which are available.

MOTOR PLANNING

Very young children enjoy marking paper with crayons or paint. Initially, there seems to be little attempt to make representations on

17

paper, the process of making marks, the movements involved and the altered appearance of the paper provide satisfaction. Maturation brings greater skill in planning movements in order to inscribe specific shapes. This mental ability to plan appropriate movements (praxis), before they are manifested on paper, is vital if drawing and writing skills are to develop. Apraxia, the inability to plan specific movements, and dyspraxia, difficulty with planning specific movements are often difficult to diagnose and understand. A person may be able to draw spontaneously a line in a particular direction but be unable to do so to command. Where handwriting is concerned, some may be able to write reasonably well when concentrating hard for a short length of time, yet handwriting in great amounts may be impossible, the writing deteriorating as it increases in amount.

DEVELOPMENT OF DRAWING SKILLS

Drawing and writing skills usually develop in a specific sequence and are acquired at certain developmental ages. Though these skills usually develop at similar ages in most children it is not abnormal for there to be some variation in the age at which they are acquired. In addition, the ability to draw specific shapes and representations of objects does not only rely on motor skills and motor planning, but also on the visual perception and understanding of them. A child's drawing skills usually develop as follows:

1. Fifteen months – imitates scribble or may scribble spontaneously when appropriate materials are familiar and available.
2. Eighteen months – scribbles spontaneously and imitates a demonstrated crayon stroke.
3. Two years – imitates a vertical stroke and round scribble. The Denver Developmental Screening Test states that to be acceptable the vertical stroke must be within 30° of the vertical (Frankenburg and Dodds, 1969).
4. Two and a half years – imitates a horizontal stroke.
5. Three years – copies a circle.
    (It should be noted that 'copy' is different from 'imitate'. 'Copy' indicates that the shape is drawn after seeing the completed shape which has not been seen in the process of being drawn, whereas 'imitate' indicates that the shape has been observed during the process of being drawn as well as when it was complete. Therefore copying a circle requires the child to

understand the shape and devise a motor plan for reproducing it. Imitating a circle requires only the imitation of the movement which was perceived during its construction.)

6. Three years – imitates a cross which is composed of a vertical and a horizontal line, not one which is composed of two diagonal lines.

Some children may attempt to draw a representation of a human figure. This may be composed of a head with some indication of features and perhaps legs (Illingworth, 1983; Sheridan, 1975). The Denver Developmental Screening Test indicates that 25% of children are able to represent a human figure with three parts at three and a quarter years and all are able to do so at the developmental age of five years (Frankenburg and Dodds, 1969).

7. Four years – copies a cross.

Representations of a human figure usually contain more parts, head, features, legs, trunk and often arms (Sheridan, 1975).

8. Four and a half – copies a square (Illingworth, 1983). Some children will imitate a square which they have watched being drawn from about three and a half years.

9. Five years – copies a triangle. This is usually the first shape children are able to draw which contains diagonal lines. This is an important milestone, for the ability to describe diagonals is necessary for the construction of letter characters and numerals.

10. Six years – copies a diamond (Illingworth, 1983). Some authorities suggest that the average age when a diamond may be drawn is seven years and that '50 per cent of seven-year-olds find imitation of the diagonal in configuration difficult to execute' (Alston and Taylor, 1987).

HAND PREFERENCE

Some babies show a preference to use one hand rather than the other between the ages of six months and one year, though this preference may change a few months later (Illingworth and Illingworth, 1984; Enstrom, 1974). This may be followed by a period of bilaterality, before the choice of preferred hand is finally established, in some children as late as four years.

There is a group of children who seem to be unable to decide on the hand with which they prefer to write, draw and paint. In a single session they may change their preference several times. This indecision regarding the preferred hand may occur when there is considerable motor deficit in both hands or when there is slight motor deficit in the hand which is innately the preferred one. Thus the child has a natural inclination to use the innately preferred hand though the other hand is the more able. Hence the trials of both hands when writing, drawing or painting. Eventually these children do decide which hand they prefer to use if they are allowed the freedom to do so. Concern is usually reduced if the reason for the delay in the development of hand preference is explained to the adults concerned.

Graham was referred for assessment by an occupational therapist a few months before his fifth birthday because his school reported that he was having problems with pencil skills. There was particular concern over his lack of progress with handwriting. His school was in the catchment area of families working at a university and consequently the standards of expected achievement within the school were higher than average.

Assessment suggested that Graham's gross motor ability was at the lower end of the normal range. The level of his performance on the left side of his body was slightly below that of the right side.

When using a pencil, Graham seemed to be equally comfortable using either his left or his right hand. Several members of his family are innately left-handed. It was thought that this indecision regarding handedness was caused by his innate left-handedness, but the motor ability of the left hand was poorer than the right.

It was suggested that Graham should be free to experiment using a pencil in either hand. It was also suggested to his parents and his teachers that, should his handwriting difficulties persist, the use of a small electronic keyboard would enable him to record on paper efficiently.

When Graham no longer felt under pressure with regard to his handedness and pencil skills he developed his left hand as his preferred one. During the following year his handwriting improved considerably and concern about his progress was decreased.

The occupational therapist suggested to his parents that should he have difficulty with the speed or legibility of his handwriting in future years, when larger amounts of handwriting will be expected from him, he should return for further assessment and, if necessary, treatment and advice.

OTHER NECESSARY SKILLS

Referring back to the developmental ages at which most children are able to produce specific effects with a pencil, the variety of skills which enable them to do so should be considered. In addition to motor and motor planning skills, many other abilities are also entailed. Sensory, perceptual and emotional elements, are also involved.

Sensory ability

Sensory ability is, of course, involved in almost all types of activity which result in recording on paper. The visual skills of focusing and scanning which develop in infancy are necessary. Perhaps the only exception being those with severe visual impairment who touch-type or use complex audiovisual equipment in order to record words. Chapter 3 describes some of the visual impairments which may impede recording skills.

Hearing is required in order to undertake such activities as note taking during a lesson or lecture, taking dictation from a teacher or perhaps writing down an address heard on the radio. These skills are not part of the motor skill of recording on paper, but are necessary if the skill is to be employed meaningfully.

Memory

A number of intellectual skills are also required for meaningful recording on paper, these include memory, both short and long term. In order to record words on paper the letter characters and their sequence within words must be remembered and readily recalled. Copy writing and typing require accurate short term memory if work is to be completed accurately. Writing material which is verbally dictated requires an accurate short term memory, in this case in the auditory, rather than the visual, mode.

Perceptual skills

Earlier in this chapter hand/eye coordination was discussed. The development of this ability entails the appreciation of self, body image, and the dimensions and relationships of body parts to each other. Throughout life, though body size, shape and proportions change, there is continuous appreciation, usually unconscious, of these dimensions.

Closely related to body image are the perceptual skills, appreciation of position in space and spatial relationships. The position of self and the relationship of the various parts of self are necessary at a gross level if appropriate positions are to be maintained and effective movements accomplished while undertaking recording tasks. Perhaps most importantly, these skills enable the hand to function effectively so that there is good hand/eye coordination.

These perceptual skills are also important with regard to the written word. Accurate appreciation of the position in space of letter characters and numerals ensures that the correct information is recorded. Many characters are similar in form but are differentiated one from the other by their position in space. Lower case p, b and d are the same shape, the differences between them being their orientation in space. Similarly, the pairs, 2 and 5, u and n, and sometimes f and t, are more or less the same shape but differently orientated. Lack of appreciation of the spatial position of letter characters and numerals can seriously impede recording skills. It should be noted that children appreciate vertical inversions before they appreciate left/right reversals. Some children are seven years old or more before they appreciate the latter. There is a greater proportion of boys than girls who experience such confusion (Chapman, Lewis and Wedell, 1970).

Motivation

Understanding of the skills required to undertake successfully the various forms of recording on paper will help to ensure that tasks and the way in which they will be accomplished are appropriate. A task successfully completed provides motivation for renewed efforts. 'When people have succeeded, they tend to feel lively and elated; when they have failed, they may be depressed and apathetic. These feelings may be prolonged' (Vernon, 1971). Thus a person's level of motor ability may make writing with a pen impractical for all but the briefest note. A keyboard may enable that person to record successfully, satisfying personal standards and aspirations. Drawing realistic pictures may not be possible, but the use of stencil or printing techniques may result in work which merits the admiration of peers and mentors, thus motivating the perpetrator to further endeavours.

3

Assessment: defining needs and problems

I keep six honest serving men
(They taught me all I know);
Their names are What and Why and When
And How and Where and Who
                            Rudyard Kipling

There are differences between assessing the abilities of children and those of adults. The young child has yet to realize his potential in all areas of development. He is not aware of what capabilities he will have in the future, what his desires will be or what opportunities he will have. Neither professionals nor parents can be certain of the speed of development or level of attainment the child will reach. Children should therefore be given as wide a range of opportunities as possible to express themselves through the written word and graphics.

Most adults, on the other hand, have usually had experience in a wide range of activities, have specific desires and know their own capabilities. When adults who have acquired disability are being assessed, past lifestyle will usually provide pointers to previous abilities and interests. Exceptions are people who have suffered congenital disabilities and may not have had the opportunity to attempt some skills, either because they are not aware of them or they have not the means to overcome disabilities. An example of such a person is Joseph Deacon who was mentioned in Chapter 1.

Because of these differences in developmental potential and life experiences, the assessment of the needs and abilities of children are therefore considered separately from those of older children and adults.

ASSESSING THE NEEDS AND ABILITIES OF YOUNG CHILDREN

The assessment of hand function and the ability to record on paper is most likely to be part of a wider range of an observation, assessment and treatment plans (Penso, 1987). Indeed it is important that this is so for, as we saw in the previous chapter, the ability to write and draw is dependent on many skills in addition to hand function.

The desire to make unique marks on paper often manifests itself as early as 15 months of age. Children with severe motor handicap will have difficulty satisfying that desire. Careful assessment of the child, his abilities and potential abilities, will often enable the child to realize that potential by the use of adapted pencils and crayons or other more sophisticated means.

Many of the disabling conditions of childhood cause multiple difficulties; it is comparatively rare to find a child who suffers from a single disability. The child who suffers from the neurological condition of cerebral palsy which affects motor ability may also have a visual or auditory deficit. The condition of spina bifida, which primarily involves sensory and motor symptoms below the level of the spinal lesion, may also result in visuo-perceptual difficulties and fine motor problems affecting the upper limbs. Therefore, when observing, assessing and planning for the maximum development of pen, pencil or keyboard skills the whole child should be taken into consideration not only the parts directly concerned with drawing and writing.

The disabling conditions of childhood are of many types.

1. Congenital and continuing, such as cerebral palsy or spina bifida.
2. Acquired and continuing, such as some forms of dystonia.
3. Acquired during childhood and in many cases resolving after a number of years, such as juvenile chronic arthritis.
4. Degenerative, such as Duchenne muscular dystrophy.

Superimposed on any disabling condition of childhood is the phenomenon of developmental potential. This potential must be taken into consideration when assessing the affects of disability on writing and drawing skills (Chapter 2). The stage of maturation the child has achieved will have a number of effects.

1. Level of maturation will affect the child's interest in different types of material which may be recorded on paper. In the earliest stages, the aim will be simply to mark paper with crayon or paint. Later, interest will develop in depicting objects and people on paper. Most children at some stage develop an interest in recording words on paper.
2. It will affect the amount and type of material teachers will expect the child to be able to record.

3. It will affect the length of the child's concentration span.

Motivation to record on paper will be influenced by past success or failure, the approval or disapproval of peers and adults.

Other disabilities will also affect the child's ability to record on paper.

Hearing deficits

These may distort both the assessment and implementation of treatment. The child who does not hear questions and instructions clearly can easily be underestimated in other areas of ability. Other children with hearing deficits may have to devote a large part of their concentration to listening to what is said to them and therefore be able to give little attention to executive skills such as drawing and handwriting.

Assessing the hearing ability of children with motor disabilities is a highly skilled and often prolonged task, for often it is necessary to condition the child to make a reliable response to sounds. It is important that the results of such tests are taken into consideration when assessing other skills in the child.

Visual deficits

These will create obvious difficulties with recording on paper if acuity is impaired. Other visual problems which may not be immediately apparent may also impair the ability to record on paper effectively.

1. Impaired visual fields will affect the child's ability to scan the whole of the writing or drawing surface unless the head is moved to compensate for the areas where the visual fields are deficient. An orthoptist or ophthalmologist should be consulted if it is thought that there is such a deficit.
2. Peripheral vision may occur in children who suffer from congenital cataracts. The child is, in effect, only able to see around the edges of the cataracts. This not only limits the area which the child can see but also makes scanning a large area a difficult and comparatively lengthy task.
3. Tunnel vision, in which the child only has vision in the central

area, limits the amount the child may see unless he or she compensates by moving the head.

4. Should the eyes not be used together, the images from each eye will not be seen as one; the image will be blurred or two images will be perceived. This condition of diplopia will affect the child's visual monitoring of what has been written.

5. Hemianopia may occur in children who suffer from congenital or acquired cerebral palsy of the hemiplegic type. One half of the visual field of each eye is affected. The child may be unaware of the problem and ignore completely either the left or right side of the work surface.

6. Nystagmus is a repetitive oscillatory movement of one or both eyes which may take place in a vertical, horizontal, rotatory or retractory direction. The degree of nystagmus may vary according to the direction or the distance of the point of fixation. Many children who suffer from nystagmus discover for themselves the angle of gaze in which there is minimal oscillation and hold their head accordingly. It is important to be aware of nystagmus when positioning a child, for the head position adopted to minimize nystagmus may not be the one usually adopted by those without this problem when handwriting, drawing or using a keyboard.

7. Visual scanning and, in the case of handwriting, the ability to scan smoothly from left to right, is important. In order to monitor visually what has been written, smooth visual saccades are necessary. Often it is not possible to remedy a visual scanning difficulty, though acknowledgement of its existence often helps the sufferer to cope with the difficulty. Parents and teachers who are aware of the problem will be able to handle any difficulties sympathetically.

8. Difficulty with accommodation, the process of adjustment of the eye to see clearly at various distances, is a condition which may affect children's ability to copy efficiently from a chalkboard onto paper because of the necessity of using distance vision to see the chalkboard and near vision to write. It may be that if accommodation of the eye to seeing near and distant objects is slow, then copying any work which is displayed at a distance will be tiring. Some children develop diverting behaviours to avoid such work. Positioning the child near to the chalkboard may help to remove some of the difficulty. Alternatively the child may be allowed to copy from the teacher's own notes which may be placed next to the copy paper on the desk or table.

Perceptual difficulties

Imperceptions of self, the relationship of self to objects in the environment and the relationships between objects can all affect handwriting ability.

Body image, the constant image we all have of the dimensions of our own body, its length, girth, the reach of arms and hands, the height the outstretched body may attain, the small space it may be bent into, is important to the skills of writing and drawing. This body awareness is for most of the time unconscious, yet we constantly use this knowledge. Body image is difficult to test in isolation though impairment of it may be observed in the children who seem to lack appreciation of their own size by trying to move into spaces too small to accommodate them. They may also not appreciate the length of limbs and their own reach in various directions. Constant self knowledge of the size and shape of the hand is necessary when writing or drawing is to be carried out effectively without frequent monitoring of the hand.

The appreciation of ones own position in space is closely related to body image. Even very young children are usually aware of their own position and do not need to visually monitor their own position before they are able to move. For example, in order to catch a ball successfully children must observe when the thrower releases the ball, judge the speed and force of the throw and arrange their hands accordingly. Normally, if appreciation of position in space is intact there will be no need to monitor visually the position of the hands in order to catch the ball successfully. This too is relevant to writing and drawing skills; the appreciation of the position of the hand is important when holding writing and drawing tools.

Position in space is also important at a finer level, particularly when writing letter and number characters of similar form which are differentiated one from the other mainly by their spatial position. For example lower case d is a right to left reversal of b.

The relationship of pen to hand and hand to paper is significant when writing or drawing. For most children the appreciation of these relationships is automatic. For those who must consciously monitor, for example, the position of their hands in relation to the pen or pencil, drawing and writing will be skills difficult to acquire. The spatial relationship of letter characters and numerals to each other is of vital importance in the written word. There is a world of difference between 19 and 91, between split and spilt. Children who must always consider the relationships of letter characters and numerals to each other will have difficulty maintaining fluent handwriting.

The ability to discriminate relevant matter from a background is necessary in all aspects of life. We must be able to discriminate both visually and auditorily. This skill is also important when copy writing either from printed material or a chalkboard. The child must be able to fix and scan the current part of the piece and not be confused or distracted by the mass of print or writing around it. A finger or a ruler may help if copy writing from printed matter next to the paper which is being written on. Some children experience great difficulty with figure/background discrimination when attempting to copy from a chalkboard when it is impossible to physically mark the point in the text they have reached.

Young children begin to learn about the constancy of the form of objects. They learn to recognize objects which are presented to them from a variety of angles as the same object. They learn to generalize and learn group terms for objects and concepts which exist in a number of forms. They understand the concepts of 'chairness', 'dogginess' etc. though these things appear in numerous forms seemingly having little in common with each other. Eventually children also learn that letter characters may be represented in a number of ways. For example e may be depicted as E, e, $\mathscr{e}$, yet each is a grapheme representing the same phoneme.

As we saw in the previous chapter, hand/eye coordination is often mentioned when discussing a child's pen and pencil skills. In order to coordinate hand and eye it is necessary for the hand to function without it being monitored by the eye. The eye must monitor what is being produced by the hand, not the hand itself. It is important to be clear what is meant by this term. In order for this coordination to occur it is first necessary to have good appreciation of body image, position in space and spatial relationships.

Poor visual memory may further complicate copy writing, for children with such problems will only be able to remember a very small number of letter characters before they need to refer again to the chalkboard. Copying will be a slow process and frequently errors will be made because of difficulty remembering graphemes and their sequence.

Other problems which may masquerade as handwriting difficulties

Children are sometimes referred for help with supposed handwriting difficulties when they have a whole range of problems only one of which is poor handwriting. Spelling difficulties, problems constructing sentences or perhaps the sequence of a piece of work may result in a child sitting with pen poised on the paper considering which grapheme to write next. Hesitation regarding the construction of a sentence can have the same result. It is surprising how many children will begin a sentence having no clear idea of how it will be completed. These hesitations can result in many unintended marks being made on the paper which can give the impression of poor handwriting *per se* should the piece of work not have been observed during its construction.

Another device which is frequently used to disguise uncertainty about the spelling of a word is to make a letter character look as if it could be one of two symbols. For example, it is 'portable' or 'portible'? The easy solution is to inscribe a letter which could be either a or i. The result, handwriting looks untidy, poorly formed and not very legible, a problem which is not primarily caused by a handwriting difficulty.

Comments may be made about a child's meagre output of written work. It is sometimes assumed that this must be due to specific handwriting difficulties. Careful observation will sometimes reveal that this difficulty is really the result of poor concentration. There will be comparatively short periods spent writing, interspersed with lengthy periods of daydreaming or attention to things other than writing.

Allan was 18 months away from his GCSE examinations. He was of average ability and assessed as capable of attaining reasonable examination results if only he could learn to write a little more quickly. It was thought that because he suffered from spina bifida it was likely that he had specific handwriting difficulties. However when his handwriting was analysed there did not seem to be any difficulties which impeded the speed of writing. His problem was diagnosed when he was observed whilst producing a piece of imaginative work. He was unable to concentrate on the task, he was distracted by interesting objects in the room, and by his own thoughts regarding things he had done in the past and planned to do in the future. His problem was one of concentration, which was treated by removing unnecessary objects from his environment. In addition he was encouraged to work with full concentration for very short spells which were gradually increased in length.

Motor difficulties

Stability

In order to have a hand, foot, mouth or other part of the body which may be used to hold a recording tool, operate a keyboard or control an electronic switch there must be stability of other parts of the body. This may be achieved by the child's own muscle tone, be assisted by appropriate seating or contrived with positioning aids such as moulded supports (Chapter 4).

Motor planning (praxis)

Before a movement may be executed it must be planned at a cerebral level. Most of this planning takes place without conscious effort. It is only when new skills are being acquired that conscious planning takes place. Thus, most movement is accomplished without conscious effort. A child making his first attempts at copying his name must give complete concentration to the formation of the letter characters. After a time the child will usually write his name without conscious effort and eventually will be able to write whatever he wishes giving little or no attention to the formation of letter characters only to the content of the piece of work. Similarly, a child learning to use a keyboard will at first give all his attention to the process of depressing the required keys. As his proficiency increases he will have assimilated the patterns of finger movements necessary in order to give his attention to the content of the piece of work he is recording.

Some children have difficulty with motor planning and though they have no impairment of movement they are hampered in their attempts to record on paper because motor planning remains at a conscious level and so the child is unable to give his attention to the subject of his recording.

Derek is employed as a garden labourer by his local council. His school career was fraught with difficulty because of problems he had with motor planning.

He was referred for assessment at a child development centre at seven years of age because he was not making progress with drawing or handwriting. He was very aware of his poor progress compared with his peers and had already developed behaviour problems.

Assessment showed that he was suffering from dyspraxia which affected both gross and fine motor ability. His treatment included practice with planning gross movement, dressing and feeding skills. His drawing skills were helped by encouraging him to copy the movements made with chalk by this therapist on a floor chalkboard. This method was chosen because kneeling on the floor provided a more stable position than sitting on a chair at a table, and both the chalk and the chalkboard are matt and provide maximum resistance. He copied movements required to form shapes rather than attempting to copy completed shapes which he did not have the motor planning ability to do.

Initial progress was good, his drawing skills improved dramatically in his first few weeks of treatment (Figure 3.1). Unfortunately this rate of progress was not maintained. Derek's behaviour problems both in school and at home continued. At nine years of age he was transferred to a residential school for children with learning difficulties. Academically he did not progress well, though his behaviour improved and today he is well established in his work in the municipal gardens.

Impairment of movement

There are many causes of movement impairment and the nature of the problem will indicate the measures which must be taken to overcome the difficulty. For some children, handwriting may never be a realistic method of recording on paper; others may experience little difficulty once initial problems have been overcome.

Some causes of difficulty with recording on paper.

Neurological

Cerebral palsy is a condition which varies in the degree of its effects. Disability may be so slight that the condition is not appreciated until the child attempts fine tasks, such as handwriting.

31

Figure 3.1: Derek's drawings at seven years of age. The small blob on the left is his first attempt to depict a human figure which was drawn during his first visit to the child development centre. The large figure was drawn after six weeks treatment aimed to help him with motor planning at both a gross and a fine level.

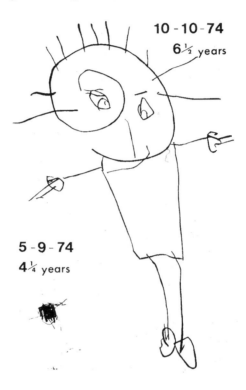

Those in close contact with the child may have noted that as a toddler the child preferred activities which did not involve precise and varied movements. Such a child may prefer to run toy cars along the floor or take a doll for a walk in its pram rather than draw or arrange small pegs in a pegboard. These preferences will most probably have been interpreted as personal taste, not as difficulty with fine motor activity.

In other children, the degree of impairment is so great that shortly after birth abnormal reflexes are observed which suggest severe impairment. Motor development is fraught with difficulty and not only is the child unlikely to develop the motor control necessary for handwriting, but the large amount of concentration and effort required to attempt to attain stability and useful movement will preclude fluent handwriting.

Tremor may be described 'as a series of involuntary, relatively rhythmic, oscillatory movements of part of the body' (Fahn, 1972). Normal tremor has a frequency of 6 cycles per second (cps) up to nine years of age, after which it increases in frequency to 10 cps by 16 years of age; by the age of 70 years the tremor has returned to the same frequency as in early childhood (Fahn,1972). Congenital tremor, also called benign essential or familial tremor, sometimes manifests itself in childhood. The tremor is clearly visible in handwriting. The effort of attempting to steady the pen or pencil is tiring for such children, who usually produce only small amounts of work and are often distressed and dissatisfied with their efforts (Figure 3.2a and b).

Dystonia may be of several forms, one of which is dystonia musculorum deformans. Following normal pregnancy and delivery, the onset of the disease is usually between the ages of 5 and 10 years (Johnson, Schwartz and Barbeau, 1962). It is characterized by abnormal involuntary movement and posturing. Handwriting is impaired by these movements when the writing hand is affected, though other grosser hand movements may be possible. The symptoms increase when voluntary movement is attempted or when the sufferer is being watched by another person.

The muscular dystrophies and atrophies result in lack of muscle power. Assessment should include ascertaining the possibility of deteriorating function as well as the expected speed of deterioration. Treatment plans should include preparing the child and his family for decrease in motor ability and providing a means of recording on paper which requires a minimum of motor effort, before that provision becomes essential. In practical terms this means the provision of a keyboard, electric or electronic typewriter or word processing element of a microcomputer, and teaching the skills necessary to use if efficiently, whilst the child is still able to write with a pen.

Children who are born with some forms of muscular atrophy will never be able to record efficiently with a pen. Such children should be introduced to keyboard skills at an early age. Maureen Goad's picture method of learning the keyboard is suitable for children who have not begun any literacy skills (Goad, 1977). Indeed the method

Figure 3.2: Alice is seven years old and suffers from congenital tremor which affects fine hand function particularly pencil skills. At a gross motor level she does not have any problems. She rides a bicycle without stabilizers, enjoys ballet lessons and has good elevation when jumping or hopping. The right is her preferred hand. a) Shows her ability to draw squares between stimulus lines using either her left or right hand. To complete the lower pair of squares she wore a weighted wrist band which slightly improved the amount of pressure exerted with the pencil on the paper and the steadiness, particularly of her right hand. b) Shows an example of Alice's handwriting at the same age. She had already discovered that very small letter characters reduced the evidence of her tremor. She found that prolonged periods of handwriting caused discomfort in her hand because of the tense posture she adopted in order to minimize her tremor. Shortly after this time she began to learn to use a typewriter with which she is now proficient and uses for long pieces of written work.

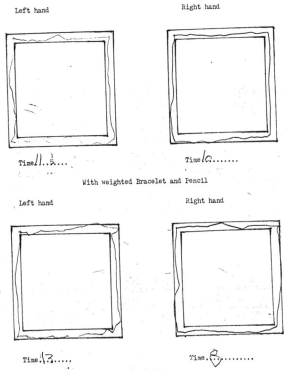

(a)

(b)

of 'colouring' pictures using one key of the keyboard in order to learn its position may also be used simply to colour simple pictures, a skill that such children could not normally undertake.

Limitation of movement

Juvenile chronic arthritis (JCA) is 'an arthritis of at least 3 months duration, starting before the 16th birthday with the exclusion of other diseases which could mimic the condition' (Craft, 1985). It describes a group of diseases which may be systemic, polyarticular (affecting many joints), pauciarticular (affecting four or less joints). The disease may continue for some years but 75–80% of sufferers are likely to have only minor or no disability 15 years after the onset of the disease (Craft, 1985). A minority of children will need adaptations to pens, pencils and paintbrushes where there is involvement of the joints of the hands and fingers. A few with continuing impairment will need to learn keyboard skills.

Arthrogryposis is a connective tissue disorder which limits the range of joint movement. There is frequently joint deformity also. These impairments vary in their intensity and the severity of the disability they cause. Arthrogryposis can cause both gross and fine difficulties which will affect positioning for recording skills and effective manipulation of tools (Figure 1.1).

Amniotic bands which may distort or cause deletion of fingers occur *in utero*. Tools with custom-made adaptations may be required in order to undertake some recording activities, though many children find their own ways of manipulating conventional tools despite the absence of some or parts of some fingers.

Syndactylism is a varying degree of webbing of fingers and/or toes which occurs in a number of conditions, one of which is Apert's syndrome. Though there may be difficulty with some very fine hand skills many children who have this condition manipulate a pen or pencil well, provided that apposition of the thumb is possible.

Minor motor dysfunction affects a relatively large number of children. These children could be described as functioning at the lower end of the normal scale of agility. The motor dysfunction may affect both gross and fine movement. Some children also have language difficulties affecting both comprehension and executive skills. As young children many prefer non-specific outdoor activity

35

to drawing and painting. Some children's difficulties may be apparent in pre-school years whereas others may not be discovered until they begin attending school, for example, poor pencil control and poor motor planning ability.

QUESTIONS TO ASK WHEN ASSESSING THE NEEDS OF CHILDREN WITH REGARDS TO RECORDING ON PAPER

What is the child's developmental level?

This should be considered rather than the child's chronological age, for the child's developmental level will indicate the level of skills in all areas of ability.

1. Gross motor skills, the ability to adopt and maintain appropriate positions will indicate the measures which need to be taken to ensure suitable positions for the practice of recording skills.
2. The level of development of fine motor skills will indicate the tools which will be suitable for recording, the types of pens, pencils and brushes, the need for adaptations or the introduction of keyboards.
3. The intellectual level of development will suggest the types of materials which the child will be able to use and enjoy using to record on paper. Though it is hoped that all children will make rapid progress with recording skills it is unrealistic to expect any child to work at full capacity all of the time. Tasks should be at a level at which success is attainable and hence motivation ensues to encourage further effort.

The answer to this question will help in deciding the aims and objectives when planning a programme to help the child.

What is the child's optimum body position for effective hand function and hand/eye coordination?

Positioning will be governed by neurological function, range of joint movement and the child's ability to maintain or be maintained in a desirable position. It should not be assumed that a sitting position is necessarily best. Some children who suffer from neurological conditions, such as cerebral palsy, have their best hand function when standing, often this necessitates the use of a standing box or frame which maintains the child in this position.

Other children may also have periods when they are constrained because of injury or surgical procedures. On such occasions special devices will be needed to secure the surface for writing or drawing. These contrived body positions will of course affect writing and drawing ability.

Pencil skills are also affected in sitting by the position of the legs. For example, children who wear long leg callipers without a knee hinge will be impaired in pencil skills because leaning forward requires flexion of the hips to less than 90°. In this position, which is adopted when sitting to write or draw, there is maximum strain on the hamstring muscles at the back of the legs when they are extended. Even callipers which do have hinges to allow knee flexion may be found to affect handwriting and drawing because of the constraint of the pelvic strap. For these reasons many fine hand activities will be best accomplished when not wearing callipers. However it is appreciated that in a classroom, where there is a rapid succession of varied activities, it is not always convenient to remove and replace callipers on a number of occasions during a school day.

How will the paper be supported?

1. Will a table be used similar to that of the peer group?
2. Will a tray be attached to a special chair or standing box?
3. Will the paper be best resting on a horizontal surface or will another angle best suit the child?
4. Will resting the hand on a sloping surface allow the child to make the best use of hand function? Will a sloping surface allow the child to make the best use of vision?

Which type of paper is most effective for the child?

A matt paper will increase friction and help to control the movement of the tool on the paper. A smooth shiny paper will facilitate the movement of tools on the paper.

Will the paper need to be secured?

This may be necessary if the other hand is unable to steady the paper. It will, of course, be very necessary if the paper is supported at an angle to the horizontal.

How important are the dimensions of the paper?

The dimensions of the paper will be dictated by the type of work being undertaken, but also by the physical abilities of the child. Limitation of arm movement will dictate the dimensions of paper unless help is constantly available to adjust its position. For handwriting purposes, writing which proceeds parallel to the longer edge of the paper will require the position of the arm, hand and paper to be adjusted less frequently than if the writing is parallel to the shorter side.

Which types of writing and drawing tools will be most suitable for the child?

Is increased friction desirable? Friction will help the child to control writing or drawing movements. It may be increased by using a matt surfaced paper and by the nature of the writing or drawing tool. Ball-tipped pens and pencils which have been much used since sharpening provide the least friction; chalk and fibre-tipped pens provide most friction.

Is movement of the writing or drawing tool over the paper difficult so that the minimum of friction is desirable?

Is the weight of the recording tool important? Would weight improve stability? Weight may be added to the writing tool itself or to the wrist of the user (Chapter 5).

Does the child lack muscle power and require the lightest possible tools and those which move over the paper most easily?

Does the grip of the tool which is possible make a special or adapted shape of tool necessary? This question is discussed further in Chapter 5.

Is the use of pens and pencils a realistic method of recording or should electric/electronic means be considered?

A child who experiences great difficulty with the mechanics of hand-writing and artwork may have to devote a lot of energy and mental effort to the practicalities of recording and have few resources available for the content of the work. Whilst peers are practising their creative drawing and writing skills, the child with motor disability is giving the greater part of effort to the mechanics of writing or drawing and thus losing valuable practice in imaginative and constructive skills. Such children benefit from the use of keyboards and electronic devices, either on a temporary basis until motor skills develop, or permanently when motor disability persists. These devices may be needed for all or part of recording activities.

ASSESSING THE NEEDS AND ABILITIES OF ADOLESCENTS AND ADULTS

The types of material which adolescents and adults wish to record on paper are different from those which young children wish or are required to record. Most adolescents are expected, in school or college, to record large quantities of words in the form of notes and essays. It is usually expected that, by this time, handwriting has become automatic; the student is able to inscribe letter characters, words and sentences without conscious regard to the mechanics of handwriting.

Adults, on the other hand, vary in the amount of recording on paper they wish or are required to undertake. Yet it is usually expected that writing will be legible, fluent and undertaken without undue regard to the construction of letter characters. Some adults use only a minimum amount of writing as a means to communication, nevertheless there are occasions when adults need to be able to write. This may only be to sign their name on cheques, forms or greetings cards. Other people are employed in situations where large amounts of handwriting are a necessary part of their job. Other occupations require the employee to type or use a word processor or microcomputer.

As discussed in Chapter 1, there is a wide range of abilities and desires with regard to the nature and quantity of material which people record on paper. There are also a large number of reasons why people have difficulties recording on paper which must be investigated before suggestions can be made to enable people to record on paper or improve their ability to do so.

Previous history

It is important to discuss the person's history of ability to record on paper if realistic recommendations are to be made. Care should be taken, however, when people, who in the past have not had the opportunity to develop recording, wish to do so perhaps because of a change in their circumstances due to disability. In such instances the reader should refer back to the section of this chapter concerned with assessment of children in addition to considering the points in this part of the chapter.

What is the nature of the disability which impairs the ability to record on paper?

1. Has the disability always been present? Was the disability congenital or occurring early in childhood?
2. Has the disability been acquired recently? If so, the person's previous ability to record on paper should be investigated. This may be difficult to elicit, for it is unlikely that an objective assessment will have been made prior to the acquisition of the disability. Clues may be gleaned from the person's educational history, past employment and general interests. Care should be taken, however, in drawing conclusions from this information, for some people may have long standing aspirations which they have been unable to realize. For example, a woman or a man may give priority to an employment which provides financial support for dependents rather than considering only personal ambitions.
3. Is the condition likely to improve? Has the disability been acquired recently and likely to resolve? Will help with recording on paper become unnecessary in the foreseeable future?
4. Is the disability the result of a degenerative condition so that manual and other skills are likely to deteriorate? Will the provision of a means to record on paper become part of adjustment to a new lifestyle as the person's physical abilities diminish? In such situations it is usually best to provide adaptations and devices before they become essential. For example, an adolescent who suffers from muscular dystrophy should learn to use a keyboard before handwriting deteriorates to such an extent that it is impracticable.

What does the person wish to record on paper?

Are the person's aspirations realistic, taking into consideration previous ability and present condition. For example, a person may have been employed as copy-typist prior to the present disability. If the only means presently available of operating a keyboard is by using a scanning device it is unlikely that sufficiently high speeds of typing will be possible for return to previous employment. Lack of speed when using such devices has been described as the stumbling block to their use (Workman, Geggie and Creasie, 1988).

1. Does present employment depend on the ability to record? Does the person need to develop recording skills because injury or deteriorating impairment makes a change of occupation necessary?

2. Is the person considering some form of recording on paper as a leisure interest? Should this be so, lack of speed will not be nearly so important as if recording skills are required in competitive employment.

3. Is it only necessary to be able to record a few words, such as a signature, a shopping list, filling in a form and the like? Will it therefore be more appropriate to find means of recording with a pen or pencil than using a keyboard?

4. Is speed of recording important? Is there a realistic means of enabling rapid recording or will aspirations need to change directions? Could, for example, recording be verbal rather than manual, using a cassette recorder rather than a pen or keyboard?

5. Are the person's expectations of recording on paper realistic? Consideration should be given not only to the physical activity of writing but also to the intellectual skills which are an integral part of any creative writing activity. Consideration should be given to the following skills:
   (a) The length of concentration span necessary to commit thoughts to paper.
   (b) Both short term and long term memory are necessary, the former to hold a sentence which has been mentally constructed until it has been committed to paper and the latter to recall the spelling of at least the vocabulary which is in frequent use. A dictionary may be consulted for words used only occasionally.

6. What financial constraints are there on the choice of method of recording? Adapting a pen is a cheap procedure; the purchase of

a microcomputer and all the other necessary items is a considerable expense. Where may help be sought for the purchase of equipment?

(a) Has the person the means to purchase equipment?
(b) Will an employer help with the purchase of equipment necessary for the person to continue in paid employment?
(c) Will a charitable organization help with funding?
(d) Are statutory funds available? Education authorities may provide special equipment which is required by adolescents and others in further education establishments. Equipment such as microcomputers which are also used to control the environment (e.g. switching a television, electric lights on and off, etc.) may be funded by social services.

Where will the recording on paper take place?

1. Will it always be undertaken in the same place? If work is always to be undertaken in the same place it is, of course, possible to use equipment which is large and heavy and such equipment may be permanently set up ready for use.
2. Is an electric outlet available? This would mean that an electric or electronic typewriter or a microcomputer may be used. Is the electric outlet in a suitable position for using the equipment?
3. Is the working position well lit by either natural or artificial light? Electric sockets are not always placed in the best positions. For example in many classrooms, the only electric socket is situated on the wall under the chalkboard, which is not a good position as far as light and seeing the chalkboard are concerned.
4. Does the equipment the person will use to enable recording on paper allow solitude should it be desired or participation within a group when appropriate?
5. Must the means of recording be portable? For example, a student in higher education will probably need to move to different rooms for each lecture or lesson, the equipment which is used to record on paper must therefore be easily portable. (Many so-called portable typewriters are moveable rather than truly portable and certainly would not be light enough to be transported by hand a number of times each day.) Equipment must not only be lightweight but also quick to pack away and set up again between each change of room. Preferably the user should be able to handle equipment without assistance.

Physical assessment

The maintenance of a stable working position is as important for adults as for children

Please refer to the section in this chapter on stability for children (p.30).

1. Is there any difficulty maintaining a suitable position for hand-writing, using a keyboard or graphic work? If overall position is no problem, probably because the impairment is confined to the hands or arms, then the general recommendations for appropriate working position should be followed (Chapter 4). Consideration should, however, be given to the length of time a particular position may be comfortably maintained.

2. Is a considerable amount of physical and mental effort required to maintain a good working position? If the person is to be able to concentrate fully on the piece of work being undertaken, the need to also concentrate on sustaining the overall working position should be removed by providing any support necessary. Other occasions should be chosen for working on stability of position.

3. Has provision of special seating already been made? Can this seating also be used when the person is recording on paper?
   (a) Is the chair or standing apparatus fitted with a suitable work surface? Is it of suitable size, height and incline?
   (b) Is it possible to use the sitting or standing apparatus with an existing work surface? Will it be necessary to design a special work surface to use with an existing chair or other apparatus?
   (c) Does the chair or standing apparatus maintain the person in a good position for working with the hands on a work surface? A chair which positions the hips at more than 90° will not hold the person in a suitable position for working with the hands on a horizontal surface, for the neck will need to be flexed in order for the eyes to monitor the work being undertaken. This position will be uncomfortable for most people, especially those with extra-pyramidal signs who may find extreme downward visual gaze painful.

   Where possible, the working position should be such that the hips are flexed to less than 90°, so that the head and hence visual gaze on the work surface is comfortable.

If it is not possible to alter the sitting position so that the above criteria are satisfied it will be necessary to alter the angle of the work surface for maximum comfort.

4. Many people with neurological dysfunction find that their hand function is best when they are in a standing position. Consideration should be given to this position and appropriate adaptations made to equipment.

Gross movement

1. Has the person sufficient independent mobility to move to and from the work area?
2. How far can the person reach? For example, can the person reach the switch of a microcomputer which is situated at the back of the machine?
3. Will special provision be necessary for the person to carry equipment?
4. Does the effort of hand movement disturb the overall position? This is likely to happen in some neurological conditions, such as cerebral palsy. If this becomes a severe problem it may be advisable to choose a means of recording on paper which requires less fine motor effort, for example using a keyboard rather than handwriting.

Hand function

1. Is it possible to hold a writing or drawing implement in the preferred hand? It is extremely difficult to become accomplished in adulthood in fine motor skills using the non-preferred hand. In the case of recording words on paper would it be preferable to use a keyboard rather than attempt to manipulate a pen in the non-preferred hand?
2. Would it be possible to hold a writing or drawing implement if it was adapted in some way? (Chapter 5.)
3. How much hand movement is possible? Are smooth precise finger movements possible? Is that movement of the type appropriate for pen, pencil and brush skills?
4. Does any involuntary movement (e.g. tremor, unsteadiness, dystonia, etc.) impair appropriate hand movement?
5. Does lack of power impair the use of tools to record on paper?
6. Does gripping or moving a writing or drawing tool cause pain or discomfort? Can this problem be removed by adapting tools? (Chapter 5.)

7. Are there motor planning (dyspraxic or apraxic) problems which impair the ability to record on paper? Though there may be little impairment of movement there may be problems with planning that movement at a cerebral level, which are particularly significant when writing or drawing where swift, varied and precise movements are necessary. A keyboard removes the need for this complex planning of movement and is often the most satisfactory solution for people with such difficulties.

8. After considering the above questions would an electric or electronic means of recording on paper be more appropriate than a pen or pencil? A microcomputer may be used not only for word processing but also for simple or sophisticated graphic work. Would the person concerned prefer to use a typewriter or microcomputer? Is the use of this type of device necessary for employment opportunities?

9. Has the person had previous experience of keyboards or will this skill need to be learned?

10. If the person has used a keyboard previously will the manner of use need to be adapted because of acquired impairment or prognosed deterioration in the user's condition?

There are many visual impairments which may hamper the ability to record on paper

Visual acuity is, of course, always a consideration. In the adult population not only the current level of visual acuity should be considered, but also the possibility of deterioration of acuity as part of the ageing process or as a symptom of the condition from which a person suffers.

Recording on paper may also be impeded by eye conditions other than imperfect acuity. These conditions include nystagmus, incomplete visual fields and problems caused by not using the two eyes together. These difficulties are mentioned in the section on assessing children in this chapter (pp.25–6).

Many questions must be asked when assessing the needs and abilities of both children and adults with regard to recording on paper. The needs of no two people are exactly the same. Skills, disabilities, aspirations and working situations all vary, so that working positions, tools, equipment and adaptations need to be considered for each individual person.

4

Positioning: people and work surfaces

Are you sitting comfortably? Then I'll begin.
Julia S. Lang, *Listen With Mother*,
BBC Radio

It is important for anyone undertaking precise work with the hands to adopt a stable overall posture, most usually in a sitting position. The body must be comfortably supported if the hands are to have their best function and full attention is to be given to the task being undertaken. The work surface must also be of a suitable size, shape and height in relation to the position of the person using it. This is applicable whether the person concerned is able bodied or has some form of motor disability. Consider, for a moment, the difference in the quality of handwriting which is undertaken in an impromptu situation, whilst resting the paper against a wall, and that undertaken whilst sitting on a suitable chair at a table; the quality of handwriting will usually be superior when the body and hand is suitably supported.

A suitable chair will be of such a depth that it supports the thighs, yet not so deep that it presses into the back of the knee. The height of the seat will allow the feet to be placed flat on the floor whilst the knee is flexed at 90° (Figure 4.1). The back of the chair will support the person's back when the hips are flexed at about 90°, though for most activities where a table is used hip flexion will be to less than 90° so that the back of the chair will not be continuously used for support.

Comfort and position will also depend on the table being used. The exact height of the table will depend on the type of work for which it is being used. Because use of a keyboard increases the height at which work is undertaken, ideally the table on which it rests should be slightly lower than one used for handwriting. Some technical drawing and other types of graphic work are carried out in a standing position which will, of course, require a higher table than one used in a sitting position.

Figure 4.1: Diagram illustrating a good basic sitting position on a chair of the correct height from the floor so that the feet may rest flat on the floor and the thighs are supported by the depth of the chair seat.

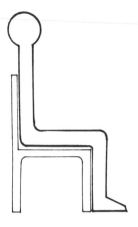

A square or rectangular work surface will provide a straight edge against which to sit and on which to rest the forearms when appropriate. Such a surface is preferable to one provided by a round or oval table, with a curved edge, which will not provide so much forearm support.

Whatever the activity, it should be possible to see, without strain, the surface on which the work is being done. Some people, for example those with extra-pyramidal symptoms, find extreme downward gaze uncomfortable and so will find a work surface which has a substantial tilt more comfortable.

In the past, almost all handwriting was undertaken with the paper resting on sloping surface, usually a desk. Many people do find that a slightly sloping surface is the most comfortable one for hand-writing. At least one teacher who has a particular interest in the development of children's handwriting, advocates the use of a padded sloping board by young children when writing (Myers, 1987).

Many secondary school students and draughtsmen use a sloping surface for technical drawing. This is appropriate for most, but not all, people. One 16-year-old boy who suffers from hemiplegic cerebral palsy finds the only surface on which he can work at technical drawing and other such activities is a flat one. Both the comfort of the person as well as the type of activity should be considered when selecting a work surface.

Taking the above points into consideration will help everyone to produce their best work when using any means to record on paper. It is particularly important to ensure a good working position for those people who have slight coordination difficulties, where overall position can make the difference between producing work of an acceptable standard and becoming fatigued after a short while and producing work which gradually deteriorates in quality.

There are also those who need specially adapted work surfaces and devices if they are to be able to record on paper at all, or to enable them to achieve their optimum standard.

ADAPTATIONS AND DEVICES

Chair height

The height of the seat of the chair must always be considered in relation to the height of the work top which will be used with it. Where a specialized work top or table must be used, it will be more appropriate to adjust the height of the chair to suit the work top than *vice versa*. This may also be the case in a classroom, where it is often preferable for children with special needs to sit at the same table as their peer group rather than be isolated by sitting at a separate table at a different height from that used by the rest of their group. The height of a chair may be adapted in a number of ways.

Extended legs

The length of the legs may be extended by screwing a second leg to them, thus increasing the height of the chair the required amount.

Chair raisers

Chair raisers may be used, into which the legs of the chair are fitted. Wooden chair raisers consist of wooden boxes into which blocks are placed of the required height. The chair legs are then placed in the boxes on top of the blocks (Figure 4.2a). Plastic chair raisers work in a similar manner, but have a fluted arrangement inside each raiser which ensures that chair legs of irregular shape may be held securely (Figure 4.2b). It is important to state that the leg which is added to increase the height of the chair should extend for the length of the original leg plus the additional amount needed to increase the height

Figure 4.2: a) Plastic chair raisers, fluted on the internal surface to hold the chair legs securely. b) Wooden chair raisers with adjustable bars which enables the raisers to be fitted to chairs of various dimensions.

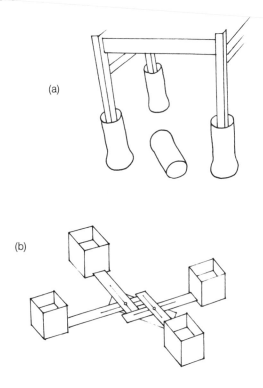

(a)

(b)

of the chair. This is to ensure that the extended leg is well supported and the chair is safe to use.

Footrests

It may be that a chair of suitable height for the work surface which is being used is too high for the user, in that their feet will not be firmly supported on the floor. This can happen with some people of restricted growth, who have a trunk of average proportions but short limbs.

The distance between the knee and the surface on which the feet rest may be reduced by fixing a footrest at the correct height to the front of the chair. In the case of a child who is growing rapidly it is advisable to attach the footrest to the chair by means of nuts and

49

Figure 4.3: a) A homemade footrest providing secure foot support where the height of the chair from the floor is too great for the user to rest their feet on the floor. b) A homemade footrest made from a wooden box of suitable height in which two holes have been cut to accommodate the front legs of the chair.

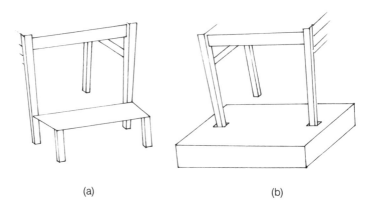

(a)   (b)

bolts so that its height may be adjusted as the child grows. The stability of the chair should be tested to ensure that it will not tip over when weight is put on the footrest whilst getting onto the chair. Should this be a problem, additional legs at the front of the footrest may be added (Figure 4.3a).

A simple adaptation to the height of a chair may be achieved using a stout wooden box which should be approximately 20 cm wider than the chair. It should measure from front to back the length of the user's feet, plus an extra 15 cm or so. The height of the box should be such that the user when sitting on the chair has their feet firmly supported on it. Two holes should be cut in the top of the box, a few centimetres from the edge that is parallel to the front of the chair, in which to fit front legs of the chair (Figure 4.3b). This type of adaptation may be quickly prepared and easily replaced, making it particularly suitable for children who grow quickly and need frequent adjustments to adaptations.

For people who suffer from tremor or other types of involuntary movements, the surface on which the feet rest may be upholstered with carpet, so that the noise of involuntary foot movements is muffled.

Arm support

Arms may be needed on a chair to provide necessary support for the person with trunk instability. The height of the arms will depend on the amount of support required; unnecessarily high support is not recommended.

For arms of the chair to provide trunk support the width of the chair seat will need to be similar to the width of the hips of the user. Chair arms may also be needed to facilitate rising from the chair. For whatever reason a chair with arms is used, care should be taken to ensure that the height of the arms does not prevent the chair being drawn sufficiently close to the table or other work surface.

Chair seat

Where there is any difficulty in maintaining posture on a chair the surface of the chair seat is important. Smooth plastic is the least suitable material. (In addition plastic chairs are frequently of rather flimsy proportions, which can make them hazardous when the person with poor motor control and lack of grading of movement lower themselves on to them.) Chairs are available which have a non-slip seat surface.

Alternatively, other chairs may be adapted by fitting them with a piece of non-slip material such as Dycem.

Sitting angle

In some neurological conditions, hand function is enhanced if the overall centre is adjusted by sitting at a slightly prone angle. The Jenx Prone Angle Chair is available in two sizes for children with a thigh length of between 60 and 215 mm. Various additions are available for children who need special support. The pronated sitting position has been found to facilitate a considerable improvement in trunk extension, head control and hand function than is possible in a conventional sitting angle. With some profoundly physically and mentally handicapped children the improvement in basic physical ability is very pleasing (Figure 4.4).

Balans seating is reported to be particularly comfortable because it encourages a straight back and trunk. The hips are at about 120°. A static version is available as well as one which is adjustable between four heights (Figure 4.5).

Figure 4.4: The Jenx Prone Angle Chair which at present is available in children's sizes.

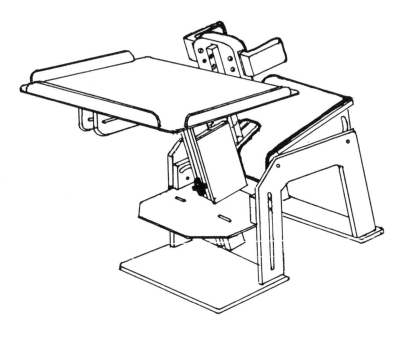

Figure 4.5: The static version of Balans seating.

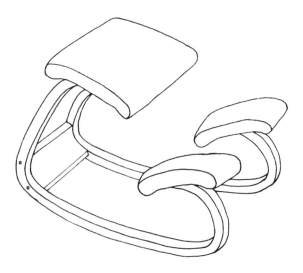

Figure 4.6: One version of an adjustable standing frame. There are a variety of models available to suit different needs.

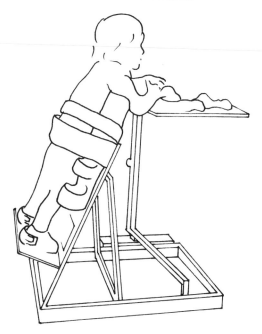

Custom-made seating

Custom-made seating will be the only type which will provide suitable positioning and comfort for some people. The provision of this type of seating requires special expertise and people are usually assessed and fitted at special centres (Rockey and Nelham, 1984; Mulcahy, 1986; Mulcahy *et al.*, 1988).

Standing

Standing may be a more functional position than sitting for some people suffering from neurological conditions. The upright position allows more effective hand function and bearing weight through the arm and hand may reduce unsteadiness of the latter. In addition, people who are not able to stand independently benefit from periods in an erect position to facilitate body drainage. Several types of standing frames and standing boxes are commercially available, it is possible to attach a work table onto most of these (Figure 4.6).

Work surfaces

The shape of work surface may need to be adapted to suit special needs. It was noted earlier that a straight edged working surface is usually preferable to a convex curve. Some children in primary schools sit at hexagonal tables, each side of the hexagon accommodating a child. With this arrangement it is not possible for six occupants to sit in a good position for drawing and writing, with forearms supported on the table, without interfering with the positions of adjacent children.

Cut out work surfaces

A work surface with a cut out which accommodates the anterior trunk will facilitate trunk position and forearm support in addition to helping maintain trunk position.

Anna, who is nine years old, suffers from spina bifida and hydrocephalus. She attends her local junior school where she moves about the classroom using a rollator. In the playground she uses a hand operated wheelchair. A full time non-teaching assistant helps with her special physical needs.

Anna is not an active child and is considerably above the desired weight for a girl of her age. Transferring from wheel chair or rollator to the chair on which she sits to work at her table is a strenuous task for her even with the assistance of her non-teaching assistant. When seated on her chair it needs to be turned towards the table and pushed near to it. Because of her size she sits on a large junior size chair which means that her feet do not reach the floor. Thus the thigh straps of her callipers cause discomfort because of the unsupported weight of the lower half of her legs. Once seated at her table her position is far from ideal! Her obesity considerable reduces the distance she is able to reach to articles placed on her table and so she needs a great deal of assistance in this area.

The advice of the occupational therapist whom she had seen before she began school was sought. She made the following suggestions:

1. A typist's swivel chair set at 90° to her table would enable Anna to transfer from her rollator or wheelchair. She could then swivel the chair round to face her table. This would remove the need for her non-teaching assistant to move Anna on her chair to face her table. In addition, when the class teacher is talking to her class from various positions in the room, Anna will be able to

turn her chair independently into a position where she can see her teacher and any apparatus she is demonstrating.

2. Providing a cut out in her table will accommodate the front of her body, thus allowing her arms to reach further across the table. It will be important to measure the position of the cut out very carefully because Anna's table abuts a wall.

3. A footrest attached to her chair would not be suitable as it would prevent Anna transferring to it, yet she clearly needs some sort of support for her feet. She is experimenting with a box, set on a piece of non-slip material which is positioned under her table and onto which she may lift her feet when in position at her table.

A cut out can also help the keyboard user who has a short trunk, where the depth of the work surface plus the depth of the keyboard between lap and flexed forearms brings the hands into too high a position. A keyboard resting on the work surface and situated over the cut out means that only the depth of the keyboard is between the user's lap and forearms.

Semi-circular work surfaces

A work surface with a cut out which also has a semi-circular outer edge will provide the largest usable surface for people who are unable to adjust their position (Figure 4.7).

Figure 4.7: A table with a cut out and curved outer edge which allows the user who has mobility difficulties to reach the maximum amount of the surface.

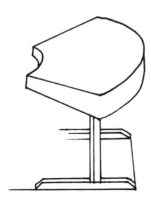

Figure 4.8: A lap desk showing a) the working surface without ledge and b) a model with ledge showing the bag filled with polystyrene beads on the undersurface.

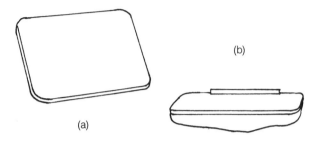

(b)

(a)

Ledges

A ledge on the outer edges of a work surface will prevent tools rolling on to the floor.

Angled work surfaces

The angle of the work surface may help or hinder handwriting, art work and even keyboard skills. Working on a horizontal surface usually means that the wrist is held in a neutral or slightly extended position. The greater the tilt of the work surface the greater the degree of wrist extension required.

Wrist extension may improve voluntary finger movement for some people. Those who suffer from some forms of cerebral palsy will find extension of the fingers easier with the wrist in extension. Thus the slope of the work surface may be a therapeutic consideration.

Lap desks

A lap desk will be suitable for some people who are confined to a wheelchair when it is not convenient to use a large fixed tray and when it is necessary to also propel the chair to different positions. Those confined to bed, perhaps because of orthopaedic conditions, may also find it useful. The lap desk is comprised of a sheet of rigid material with a plastic surface, to the underside of which is attached a fabric bag filled with polystyrene balls. This malleable undersurface allows it to mould to the users lap. It may also be moulded into suitable positions for use on a bed, including one which slopes down towards the user. It thus provides an easily portable, stable writing or drawing surface. Its usefulness though, it limited by its size (approximately 50 × 30 cm) (Figure 4.8). Commercially available lap desks often have a ledge along one long side. This is presumably to provide a rest for writing tools and to prevent them rolling off it. However its position is rather inconvenient for the hand whilst writing or drawing and it may be appropriate to reverse the desk so that the ledge is on the side furthest away from the user.

Easels

An easel may provide a suitable working position for some people, not only for painting and drawing but also for handwriting. When working on an upright, or almost upright, surface there will be greater extension of the wrist than when working on a horizontal one. Visual gaze will be in a mid position which will be more appropriate for people who find downward gaze uncomfortable. It may also be more comfortable for those with tunnel vision. The exact angle of the work surface will need to be very carefully arranged to suit the user. Care should also be taken to ensure that the easel is stable, particularly if the user will exert any degree of pressure on it. There should certainly be a substantial wooden or metal stay between the back and front parts of the easel; chain or rope will not provide sufficient stability.

Microcomputer trolleys

Access to microcomputing equipment can be difficult for people who use some special types of chairs. Chair arms may prevent the chair being drawn sufficiently close to a conventional trolley. Immobility may prevent the user reaching all the controls of conventionally arrayed equipment. A conventional trolley also dictates the height of the chair which must be used which is not always appropriate for people with disabilities. A custom-made trolley will often overcome all these difficulties if it is designed so that the height and tilt of the keyboard may be adjusted and the monitor position can also be adjusted so that it is accessible should it be used with a touch screen (Osborne, 1978).

Grips

Stability and function in the hand being used for drawing or handwriting etc. may be further enhanced by providing a grip for the

Figure 4.9: a) A work surface with a vertical post to be gripped by the left hand. b) A work surface with a horizontal bar suitable for gripping with either the left or the right hand.

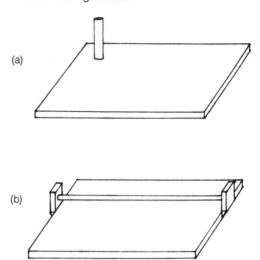

other hand usually positioned so that the arm is extended. If the best grip is in a vertical position a post of suitable diameter to provide a comfortable grip should be provided. A bar set above the working surface will facilitate a horizontal grip (Figure 4.9).

Paper

The type of paper used for recording by manual means can, to some extent, affect output.

1. The quality of the paper, whether rough, matt or shiny, will affect the manner in which the recording tool moves over it. Those people who have difficulty controlling hand movements will benefit from using paper with a matt or slightly textured surface. Those who have difficulty with initiating or sustaining movement may find that a slightly shiny surface is best.
2. The size of the paper used will depend on the range of hand and arm movement possible as well as the nature of the work being undertaken.
3. The orientation of the paper for handwriting may also be

significant should there be limitation of movement. Paper arranged so that writing is parallel to the long side of the paper will reduce the amount of adjustment which will need to be made to the position of the paper as more lines of writing are completed.

(For methods of securing paper, see Chapter 6.)

The working position

Working position makes a difference to hand function, particularly for people with motor disabilities. Ensuring the optimum working position provides the basis for making the best use of writing and drawing equipment, typewriters and microcomputers.

5

Pens, pencils and brushes

The pen is the tongue of the hand – a
silent utterer of words for the eye.
Henry Ward Beecher, *Proverbs from*
Plymouth Pulpit (1887)

A variety of tools may be used to record on paper, some of which
are dictated by the nature of the task to be undertaken. There are
times when the choice of tool will also be influenced by the abilities
and disabilities of the user. For example, a felt-tipped pen will be
more easily controlled by the unsteady hand than one with a ballpoint. Techniques other than marking paper directly with pen, pencil
or brush will help people with motor planning difficulties produce
more satisfying art and graphic work (Chapter 6). Being aware of
the range of tools which is available and their qualities will help in
making the best choice for both the task being undertaken and the
abilities of the user.

PENCILS

The part of the pencil which marks the paper may be made of a
number of materials (e.g. graphite, analine, charcoal). The graphite
(sometimes still referred to as the lead, because pencils used to be
of this material) may be of varying degrees of hardness which is
denoted by a mark on the pencil: 2H is very hard, 4B is very soft,
HB is midway between the two. Usually the purpose for which the
pencil is to be used dictates the hardness of the graphite chosen. For
free drawing a soft pencil is usually used for outlines and shading.
A hard pencil is used for technical drawing, where a fine accurate
line is required. An HB pencil is suitable for handwriting.

   For people who have motor disability, not only the hardness of the
pencil which is usually employed for a particular task must be
considered, but also the abilities and limitations of the user. People
who are only able to exert light pressure on paper will mark the

Figure 5.1: a) A pencil sharpened with a pencil sharpener where the graphite and the wood is shaped to a fine point which is liable to breakage should heavy pressure be applied. b) A pencil sharpened with a penknife where the sharpened area is less acute and a smaller area of wood is removed.

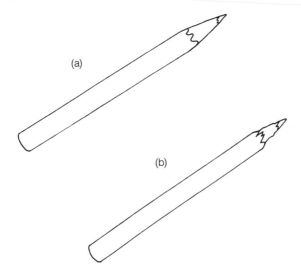

paper more effectively with a soft pencil. Those who are unable to grade the amount of pressure they exert may prefer a slightly harder pencil than would normally be used.

A freshly sharpened pencil will provide a fair degree of friction against the paper though the point will be worn down quite rapidly, decreasing its frictional properties. A hard pencil will retain its fine point for longer than a soft one. Care should be taken when sharpening pencils: often it will be appropriate to use a penknife rather than a pencil sharpener, because the former will allow more choice in the length of graphite which will be exposed and the amount and angle of the wood which remains to support the graphite. Exposing only a small amount of graphite and leaving plenty of wood to support it is important when the pencil will be used by a person who applies heavy pressure (Figure 5.1).

Retaining a good point on pencils is often a problem for young people who have general coordination problems. They frequently have difficulty with producing legible and even handwriting at speed, maps and diagrams, as well as general difficulties with the presentation of work. Stressing the importance of having well sharpened pencils at all times can make a difference to the appearance of work. Making a habit of regularly sharpening pencils helps.

The barrel of the pencil may be cylindrical, hexagonal or octagonal, triangular or square. A shape should be selected which suits the user. A cylindrical one allows it to be used in the position in which it is picked up and requires no adjustment of the position of the fingers. Many-sided barrels may be uncomfortable for people who have tender skin, or painful interphalangeal joints. A triangular shaped barrel accommodates the thumb on one side, the index finger on the other and the lateral side of the middle finger on the third side. Whilst these triangular pencils encourage a tripod grip, the position of the thumb and index finger may be uncomfortable for some people because these two digits are very closely apposed near the apex of the triangle.

The diameter of the barrel is also significant: the smaller the diameter the closer will be the apposition of the thumb, index and middle fingers. Clearly those who find apposition uncomfortable, painful or limited by joint restriction will find a pencil barrel of larger diameter more comfortable. It should not be assumed that all young children will work best with a thick pencil. 'Certainly children show a preference for rather thinner than average writing tools when left to choose for themselves. In general, as with all learning activity, a wide experience of different media is usually most helpful to development' (Jarman, 1984).

Pencils may be made of natural unpolished wood, finished with paint or a plastic coat each providing a varying degree of friction. The more matt the surface the greater the friction and there is less likelihood of it slipping whilst it is being held to draw or write.

A propelling pencil, in which lengths of graphite are encased within a tapering metal or plastic barrel, may help the independence of people who are unable to sharpen a pencil themselves. The mechanism whereby fresh graphite is exposed should be examined and a type chosen which may be activated by the intended user. Milling on the part to be turned to expose fresh graphite will enhance the user's grip on it.

Another aid to independence is a pop-a-pencil. The tool consists of a number of pieces of graphite each of which is enclosed in a very short plastic barrel. A number of these barrels fit one into the other so that when new graphite is required the used barrel is removed to expose a new one with fresh graphite. The used barrel is replaced at the other end of the tool thus maintaining its length.

Pencil grips

It is possible to adapt the barrel of a pencil in a number of ways to suit the user, either with a commercially available grip or one which has been made for an individual user.

1. Triangular pencil grips are available in sizes to fit a standard pencil and those with a barrel of greater diameter. They are made of matt-surfaced plastic which has a soft feel (Figure 5.2b). These grips may be of help in several ways:
   (a) They are softer than the pencil itself and therefore comfortable to hold, particularly for the user who adopts a rather firm, tense grip.
   (b) When accurately positioned, they provide an indication of the position on the barrel of the pencil which should be gripped. Some children develop the habit of either gripping the pencil too near the tip or too high up the barrel. In these instances the grip indicates the correct position of the fingers.
   (c) They prevent a round pencil from rolling out of reach of the user. An important point for those who cannot adjust their position independently, stretch or reach down to the floor.
   (d) The three sides of the grip provide specific places for the thumb, index and middle fingers to form a tripod grip. For some people the short term use of such a grip results in a permanent improvement in pencil grip.
   (e) They increase the diameter of the pencil barrel slightly, which for some people is an added advantage.
2. Another type of pencil grip is available similar to the one described above, which has dimples to accommodate the thumb, index and middle fingers in the appropriate positions. Some users feel that the positions of the dimples allow the fingers to adopt a more natural position than the grip which is of a basic triangular shape.
3. Grips similar to those which are commercially available may be fashioned exactly to the needs of the user from thermoplastic material primarily intended for splinting. This material becomes malleable in hot water and may be refashioned a number of times. There is a tendency for it to stick to the barrel of the pencil and when forced up the pencil barrel to facilitate sharpening, to become a loose fit and so require remodelling.
4. A suitable length of sponge rubber tubing may be used as a grip for pencils as well as for other tools. It is available in various

Figure 5.2: a) A pencil with weight added to the end by the addition of a hollow novelty trim which has been filled with modelling clay. b) A pencil to which a triangular grip has been added to encourage a dynamic tripod grip and to indicate the position on the barrel of the pencil where it should be gripped. c) Two crayons taped together with non-allergic surgical tape, providing a quickly constructed T-shaped crayon for those who draw using a horizontal whole hand grip.

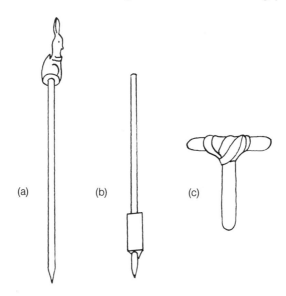

(a)   (b)   (c)

diameters and bores. There is also choice regarding the firmness of the foam. It is therefore possible to choose tubing suitable for a large range of writing and drawing implements which is also of appropriate diameter and firmness for the user. It is purchased in lengths which are cut to the desired size (Figure 5.3a).

5. A ball with an appropriately sized bore across the diameter will provide a grip for a pencil for those unable to adopt a conventional tripod grip. The size of the ball used will be dictated by the size of the user's hand and the degree of flexion in which it is most comfortable to hold the fingers. The material of which the ball is made will again be dictated by the needs of the user (Figure 5.4).

(a) Polystyrene may be useful for those with little muscle power because of its lightness, though this material is not durable and may need frequent replacement.

(b) A rubber ball of appropriate size may also be used. A solid

Figure 5.3: a) A fibre-tipped pen to which a commercially available foam rubber grip has been added. b) A paint brush which has been fitted with foam rubber tubing. Either of these grips will help those with limited finger flexion to grip tools effectively. Their matt surface and resilience helps to prevent the tool from slipping.

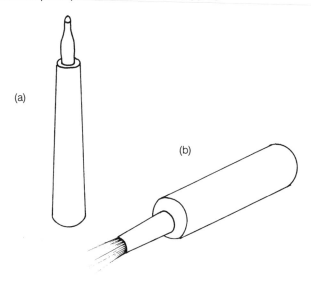

(a)

(b)

Figure 5.4: A pencil fitted with a ball to use as a grip where a thumb and four finger grip is most effective.

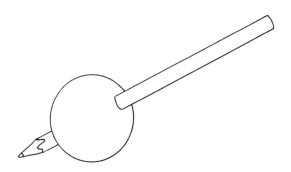

Figure 5.5: Commercially available foam grips which are shaped to accommodate the thumb and finger.

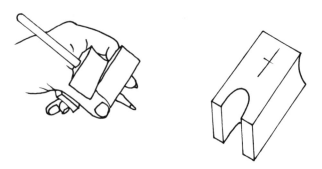

rubber ball will provide maximum weight where desirable. An alternative means of adding weight to this type of grip is to use a hollow ball into which fisherman's weights are placed before inserting the pencil (Figure 5.4). The use of these grips is not, of course, limited to pencils, they may also be used with pens, brushes and other tools.

6. Foam rubber grips with a slit to accommodate the writing tool and concavities in which the fingers are placed are helpful for people who find apposition of the thumb and fingers limited by joint restriction or pain (Figure 5.5).

PENS

Usually a pen will be more suitable tool for handwriting than a pencil. Many types of pen are available and choice should, of course, be made according to the needs of the user.

Pens are available which cost a few pence or many pounds. Choice will be governed to some extent by the financial means of the user.

The weight of the pen is governed by the material from which it is made. A pen with a plastic case it lighter than one which is made from certain metals. A lightweight pen will suit those with limitation of muscle power. A heavier pen may help those with tremor or other hand instability.

The texture of the material from which the barrel is made will affect how the pen is held. A very smooth material will require a firm grip to maintain the desired position. Pens are available with a barrel formed of non-slip material. Not only will this make the maintenance of the appropriate grip easier but this material has a soft feel which will be suitable for people with sensitive skin. It is, of course, possible to apply non-slip material to the portion of the barrel of a pen which is gripped, though this material does not have the pleasant feel of that used on purpose-made non-slip pens.

The diameter of the barrel of the pen is often a matter of personal preference. Some people feel that they have better control when using a pen with a barrel of a particular diameter. People with limited finger flexion will probably enjoy using a pen with a barrel of large diameter.

Types of pen

Many types of pen are available, the writing points of which provide a greater or lesser degree of friction and pliability. The type of pen chosen will, of course, vary according to the needs of the user. A person who has difficulty controlling the movement of the pen will manage better with one which provides a degree of friction against the paper. For those who have difficulty with initiating or sustaining a flow of fine hand movement, a pen which exerts little resistance to movement over the paper will probably prove effective.

Ballpoint pens

Ballpoint pens provide a minimum of friction; their tip is a ball bearing which is designed to reduce friction. The writing points of these pens vary in fineness. Generally it is less easy to control the precise movement of a ballpoint than other pens and so their use by school-children is usually not encouraged. However, people who have difficulty initiating or sustaining the movement of a pen may find a ballpoint the best type to use. It should also be noted that a ballpoint pen must usually be held at a more vertical angle in order to bring the writing point in contact with the paper than is the case with other types of pen.

Some of these pens have caps which cover the writing tip when not in use, others have a writing tip which may be retracted by pressing a button at the non-writing end of the pen or a clip which can also be used to secure the pen to a pocket in clothing, a handbag or briefcase. A third method some pens use for retraction is twisting one part of the barrel against the other. For some people replacing a cap may be difficult and retracting the tip by pressing the securing clip or twisting the barrel equally so. Retraction by means of a button at the non-writing end may be preferable because it can be pressed on a hard surface to do so.

Fountain pens

Fountain pens are perhaps not used so much today as in the past, yet a wide variety of these pens are still available. One of the main advantages of a fountain pen is that it provides a fair degree of friction and it is therefore easier to control the movement of the writing tip than it is with a ballpoint pen. Usually rather indifferent handwriting appears to have more character when a fountain pen is used.

Few fountain pens today have a reservoir which is filled from a bottle of ink, most use cartridges of ink. Though this method of refilling the pen is easier than filling from a bottle of ink it is not without hazards and requires a good deal of fine finger movement. There are now a number of fountain pens which are disposable and are replaced with a new pen when the ink supply is exhausted. These pens would be particularly suitable for people who write best with a fountain pen but find replacing the ink cartridge difficult.

The nibs of fountain pens vary in size, the amount of nib which is exposed, pliability, the width of the writing tip and the angle at which it is cut. If an angled, broad nibbed pen is used care should be taken to choose a pen which is correctly angled according to the hand which is used for writing.

All fountain pens have a cap which protects the nib when not in use. Caps may either push or screw onto the pen. The method of securing the cap should be considered in relation to the user's hand skills if the pen is intended to be used entirely independently.

Fibre-tipped pens

Fibre-tipped pens are available with writing tips of various shapes and diameters including those intended for handwriting. Fibre tips provide a good degree of friction and are therefore easy to control. They move smoothly on the paper and have a softer feel than a metal writing tip. They may not be suitable for people who exert a great deal of pressure when writing as the writing tip will soon be spoiled. Conversely, people who are able to exert only very light

Figure 5.6: The Biocurve pen

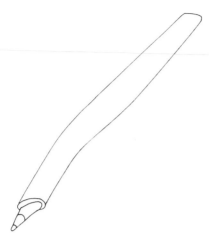

pressure on the paper will find that a fibre tip readily marks the paper effectively.

Nylon and plastic-tipped pens

Nylon and plastic-tipped pens are usually designed to produce a fine line. Their tips are more durable than fibre tips and their fineness is retained. However the writing point is not flexible and some people may find them uncomfortable to use for prolonged periods of writing.

Adapted pens

1. The Biocurve pen is contoured to fit snugly in the hand. It has wide sides which gives a larger area to grip. It has been found to be a good shape for people who need to use the non-writing hand to steady the writing because its curves cause the pen to exert less pressure on the writing hand (Figure 5.6).
2. For people who suffer from unsteadiness of the hands, an adaptation which requires downward pressure may be helpful. This pressure may be increased by using the adaptation in a standing position thus bearing downward pressure through the entire arm.
   (a) A device is commercially available which requires only a whole hand grip and may, if necessary, be controlled by arm

Figure 5.7: Writing device for people who can only adopt a whole hand grip. Because downward pressure is applied it may help those who have a degree of unsteadiness to produce firmer strokes when writing.

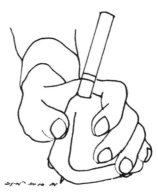

and shoulder movement. The triangular base of the device is fitted with three ball bearings so that it moves easily over the paper (Figure 5.7).

(b) The Steady Write pen is a commercially available device in which the pen is held at a writing angle by the hypotenuse of a triangle which is attached to a base which is pressed by the writing hand onto the writing surface. The user holds the device not the pen. It is reported to be helpful for people who have unsteadiness of the writing hand or limitation of movement (Figure 5.8).

3. A pen holder may be fashioned from wire for use by people who have little or no finger flexion. A coil of wire holds the pen in place. This coil is attached to a second piece of wire which encircles the proximal phalanges (Figure 5.9).

4. For the hand which is able to move adequately to form letter characters but has difficulty maintaining the grip of the pen a small splint/pen holder may be made using thermoplastic material. The splint should be made which encloses the distal part of the thumb and index finger with the pen secured between them.

5. A mouth stick with an attachment will allow limb deficient or paralysed people to draw, paint or write. The stick will be custom-made to suit the needs of the user; how the stick is held in the mouth and the relationship of the mouth to the writing

Figure 5.8: The Steady Write pen.

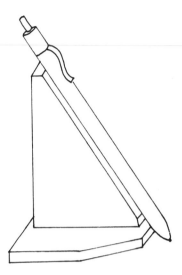

Figure 5.9: A wire pen or pencil holder which may be adjusted to suit the hand and writing or drawing angle of the user.

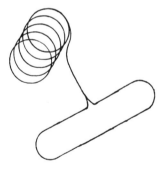

drawing or painting surface. The attachment which holds the recording tool will also vary according to the type of tool which is being held. The attachment may be a blind tube or a two piece cylinder which clamps together. Attachments are usually custom-made to suit the individual user and the recording media which will be used (Nelham, 1988).

71

BRUSHES

As with pens and pencils, many brushes are designed for a specific use. For people with manipulation difficulties some brushes may be easier to handle than others. A brush which has long soft bristles will be unsuitable for people who are unable to grade the amount of pressure they use when painting. A brush with short bristles will be easier to control and should either be purchased as such or the bristles may be trimmed so that they are of suitable length.

For similar reasons, a brush with coarser, and hence stiffer, bristles may be more easily manipulated than one with finer more pliable bristles. A stubby stencilling brush will provide maximum resistance where there is difficulty grading the amount of pressure which is applied to it. Such a brush will be best used by holding it almost vertically in relation to a horizontal work surface. This will be an ideal working position for people whose best grip is with the whole hand in a vertical plane. Many of the suggestions made about pens and pencils may also be applied to brushes. Similar devices may be used to adapt the area of the brush handle which is gripped. Where a slim handled brush requires an adapted grip the original handle may need extra padding before a commercial grip may be securely attached.

Adding a gripping bar which makes the brush handle into a T-shape will enable it to be used by people who use a whole hand horizontal grip (Figure 5.10).

Consult the following chapter for alternative methods of applying paint.

Figure 5.10: Two examples of T-sticks used for applying paint. Left, a paint brush, the handle shortened and a T-bar added. Right, a dowel T-stick with a foam rubber painting pad; foam tubing is added to the T-bar to facilitate a more comfortable, secure grip.

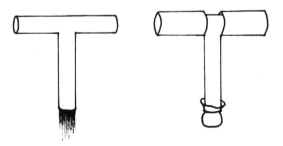

6

Tools and techniques for artwork

Art distills sensation and embodies it
with enhanced meaning in memorable form
– or else it is not art.
Jacques Barzun, *The House of Intellect*
(1959)

Artwork covers a vast range of skills and techniques. It may be a child's first attempt to apply colour to paper, a sophisticated picture by skilled artist, a rough diagram to describe the roads to be taken to a specific destination, or a precise technical drawing of a device or process. Most people at some time in their life wish or need to produce some form of artwork.

People wish to learn techniques, develop them or regain them. The process of learning art techniques begins in childhood. Most young children enjoy applying colour to paper by means of paint, crayons and felt-tipped pens; today they also enjoy novelty techniques such as pens with invisible ink, metallic or day-glo effects. Older school age children learn to manipulate rulers, set squares, protractors and compasses. They also learn printing techniques, potato and lino cuts, screen printing and tie dyeing. Some children, because of motor disability, will be limited in the types of artwork they are able to undertake, or from which they may gain satisfaction knowing that they have produced a finished product commensurate with their aspirations. For some children with motor disability, it may be preferable to use alternative techniques to drawing with a pencil or crayon or painting with a brush. Should a child's disability prevent production of artwork which satisfies the child and if their artwork is not comparable with that produced by the peer group, it will be better that the child uses other techniques with which work may be produced to a satisfying standard.

Nicholas first attended a child development centre during his first year, because of motor delay. Subsequently he was found to suffer from severe comprehensive, expressive and articulatory language difficulties. He also had slight visual problems. He therefore attended for speech, occupational and physiotherapy on a regular basis and was under the supervision of an orthoptist.

He made good progress and benefited from the many hours of patient help his parents devoted to him. All the strategies and techniques suggested by his therapists were reinforced at home. He was able to attend his small rural primary school where he received sympathetic help from his teachers. Though his motor ability had improved he continued to have great difficulty with pencil skills. However, he readily adapted to the use of an electric typewriter for written work, and a scheme for providing reconditioned typewriters for people with disabilities, which was in operation at the time, enabled him to have a second typewriter in his home.

His main problem in school was now drawing and painting. He was far from satisfied with his efforts, which looked like those of a pre-school child when his chronological age was seven years. His problem was partly solved by introducing alternative artwork using stencils, printing and rubbing techniques. Nicholas, now twelve years old, is developing an interest in microcomputers which should provide means whereby he is able to create graphs and charts as well as graphics.

Adults may have lost the ability to undertake artwork because of acquired motor disability. This artwork may have been undertaken as a hobby, semi-professionally providing a supplement to a main income or professionally. These people will, if possible, welcome the provision of means whereby they may continue to use their skills. Such skills may have taken on even greater importance to the person if the motor disability prevents them from carrying on their usual occupation. It may be important to them as a means of supplementing their income, which may already be reduced because of disability, and also as a means to occupy long days of inactivity and, perhaps most importantly, to boost self-esteem and give a *raison d'etre*.

Following the years of formal education, apart from drawing impromptu diagrams to clarify verbal descriptions, many people have no interest in any form of artwork. The development of motor disability may limit activities which have previously been of interest.

Such people may then show an interest in developing their artistic skills with brush, pencil or other means.

To enable people with motor disability to undertake artwork it is necessary to be aware of the range of tools and equipment which is available and it may be necessary to adapt tools with which they are already familiar or to introduce them to new techniques.

PENCILS AND PENCIL CRAYONS

The types of pencils which are available and the types which are suited to people with particular disabilities are described in Chapter 4. A description of the various types of home-made and commercially available grips is also given.

For drawing, a soft pencil is usually the most suitable. For technical drawing, where fine precise lines are required, a harder pencil is used which may be sharpened to a fine point. Exceptions may have to be made to these rules so that some people may use a pencil which they can handle more easily.

Various qualities of pencil crayons are available. Such crayons are encased in a wooden barrel making them the most suitable colouring medium for people who have difficulty grading the firmness of their grip or who frequently drop them on the floor; breakage is less likely than the wax crayons. With a pencil crayon it will be easier to obtain a fine point for filling in detail. Some pencil crayons are produced in blendable colours, thus allowing the user to increase the range of shades which are available from a limited number of pencil crayons. The barrel of a pencil crayon is firmer to hold than some other types of crayon and is less likely to be broken by those who have a strong grip.

CRAYONS, CHARCOAL, CHALKS AND FELT-TIPPED PENS

The choice of type of crayon should be made to suit the needs of the user with regard to the diameter of the barrel and the degree of friction produced at the point of contact between crayon and paper. Some types of crayon are heavier than others and the choice will then be made according to whether the user benefits from weight in order to gain stability or the user lacks power and needs the lightest tool possible.

Pastel colours

Pastel colours have a fine chalk-like texture. Ones hands easily become soiled when using them and they are relatively expensive to buy. However, they mark paper with little effort and when applied to paper the colour may be smudged for special effects. Two or more colours may be used on a single area of the paper and blended together. Pastel colours are particularly effective when applied to heavily grained paper. The combination of the matt surfaced pastel colour and textured paper is particularly suitable for people who benefit from added resistance. Another advantage of pastels is that, unlike chalk, they do not produce dust.

Wax crayons

Wax crayons are available in a variety of shapes and sizes. Some are slimmer than an average pencil, others are as much as 1.5 cm in diameter, which also usually means that they are weightier than the slimmer variety. Wax crayons are also available which are short and fat. Slim wax crayons are also available which have a plastic coating which helps to prevent the breakages which often occur in normal wax crayons. The wax drawing surface of these crayons is usually very smooth and therefore provides little resistance against the paper. This may preclude their use by people who have difficulty controlling and grading movement. Wax crayons are often the first type of drawing tool given to young children. However, they are not always the most suitable drawing tools for children who have motor disability; in many instances a tool which provides more friction is more suitable.

The drawing points of wax crayons quickly become blunt with use; constant sharpening is necessary to maintain a tapered point and this makes them unsuitable for fine line drawing.

Fluorescent crayons

Crayons in fluorescent colours may increase motivation to attempt drawing and designing for some people, particularly children. Their fluorescence may help people with decreased visual acuity to monitor their own progress on the paper.

Metallic crayons

Metallic coloured crayons may be used to add highlights to work. Thick metallic crayons produce rich effects when used for brass rubbings or rubbings of other designs in relief.

Aqua crayons

Aqua crayons may be used dry or with water. Used dry they have an effect similar to ordinary crayons; when dipped in water their effect is similar to painting sticks. They are available 1 cm in diameter and a thicker version 1.5 cm diameter.

Face paints

Face paints which are non-toxic and wash off with soap and water are available in both 1 cm and 1.5 cm diameters. They are useful as an aid to teaching the parts of the face and their names, the colour drawing attention to them.

Fabric crayons

Fabric crayons, which may be used to add decorative effects to clothing and household textiles, are available in several types. One type is first used to draw a design on paper, which allows any number of experiments to be made before committing it to fabric. When the desired design is completed on paper, it is then placed design side down on to the fabric and fixed onto the fabric by ironing. This type of crayon is only permanent on synthetic fabrics.

Another type of fabric crayon allows the design to be drawn directly onto the fabric and fixed by ironing. There are crayons of this type which are permanent on both synthetic and natural fabrics.

A third type of fabric crayon is removable by washing. These crayons are intended to mark designs on fabric which will later be embroidered or appliqued. They may also be useful for experimenting on natural fabrics before applying permanent crayon or paint.

Charcoal

Charcoal, which readily marks paper with the lightest touch, is available in a number of forms. Sticks of charcoal, the actual twigs which have been charred, come in a variety of lengths. They are fragile and crumble unless handled carefully. They are not suitable for people who are unable to grade their grip and release. Compressed charcoal sticks are stronger than traditional charcoal. They are available in various shades of grey.

Many people will find a charcoal pencil easier to handle. This is a charcoal core encased in a wooden barrel. It is therefore much cleaner to use because there is no need to handle the charcoal and it is obviously less liable to break. It will also be a simple matter to fit a special grip should this be required.

Chalks

Chalks may be primarily intended for use on a chalkboard or they may be specially prepared for use on paper or other surfaces when they are more properly called pastels. The nature of these chalk and chalk-like materials make them especially suitable for use by people who benefit from added friction. Chalk has a very matt surface which provides a degree of resistance in use.

Though most chalk is described as 'anti-dust' and is certainly less dusty than chalk used to be, it still gives off some powdery residue in use which may exclude its use by those who are sensitive to dust. Chalk is also fairly brittle and breaks if not treated gently. It would not be suitable for people with little grading in the power of their grip.

When used on a chalkboard, the chalk together with the matt surface of the chalkboard provides a high degree of resistance and friction. Drawing on a chalkboard, of course, is not a permanent means of recording; however it is a very useful medium for children who have poor fine motor control or a problem with motor planning (dyspraxia). This is especially so if the chalkboard is placed flat on the floor so that the child kneels down in front of the board. In this position the child is more stable because more of his body is in contact with a firm surface than would be so if sitting on a chair. If a large chalkboard is used, a second person may kneel beside the child and demonstrate the chalk strokes to be made, thus the child has a demonstration of exactly what he must do. This is much more effective for the dyspraxic child than showing him a completed example of a drawing, for the nature of dypraxia is such that there is understanding (perception) of the shape, letter character etc. but difficulty with planning the movements necessary to execute it.

Sometimes the fact that a drawing on a chalkboard is not intended to be permanent is also an advantage for the person who is nervous about attempting to draw and afraid of making mistakes. Such a person may hold the chalk in the drawing hand and a duster or chalkboard rubber in the other, so that mistakes or anything which does not satisfy may be immediately erased. This strategy often helps to build self-confidence in the ability to draw.

Chalks may also be used to draw on paper; heavy, coloured, matt sugar paper (construction paper) being the most suitable. More suitable for using on paper, however, are pastels. They are considerably more expensive than chalks, though there are cheaper versions of oil based pastels which are intended to be used by children. These are thicker than the more usual pastels which may make them suitable for people of all ages who manage a thicker tool more easily.

Felt-tipped pens

Felt-tipped pens mark paper with the minimum of pressure and so are suitable for use by people who lack muscle power (Figure 6.1). They are available with tips of various thicknesses so they may be used for a number of purposes. Because of the nature of their tips they provide a fair degree of friction especially when used on matt surfaced paper which makes their movement on the paper easy to control. A disadvantage is that very heavy pressure will easily spoil the tip. Their colours are usually clear and bright which makes them suitable for use by those with impaired vision.

Care must be taken to replace the caps immediately after use to prevent the pens drying. This need to frequently remove and replace the caps can make them difficult for some people to use. The caps usually pull off and need to be pressed on, often difficult movements for those with poor muscle power, lack of fine finger movement or the use of only one hand. Caution is required where the user may attempt to remove caps with the mouth; children often do so. There is a danger that the cap may accidentally lodge in the throat. One way to ensure that this cannot occur is to prepare a holder for the pens into which the caps are securely glued. The caps are then replaced on the pens by pressing them into the holder which contained the caps.

Figure 6.1: Two pictures by the same girl whose handwriting is shown in Figure 1.1. She drew the pictures, when she was 6 and a half years old, using felt-tipped pens held in the cleft between her index and middle fingers. Note the degree of fine control she has of the pen enabling her to draw very accurately and add so much interesting and amusing detail.

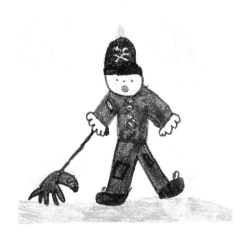

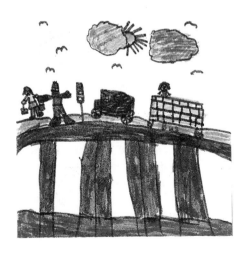

Figure 6.2: An eraser held in a bulldog clip which provides a larger, firmer area to grip.

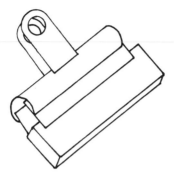

ERASERS

Most people at times wish to erase or make corrections to their work. A number of types of eraser are produced which are intended for removing marks made by specific drawing tools. Whenever possible it is sensible to use the type of eraser intended for the removal of a particular type of mark. However, many people with impaired hand function will be able to handle one type of eraser better than another. The more dense erasers are intended for removing pencil marks and soft putty erasers for removing pastel and charcoal marks. Different sizes of eraser are also available; generally the larger ones are easier to handle. Those on which one end is chamfered allow the accurate erasure of a small area, particularly when that area is surrounded by one which is not to be removed.

Some people will manage an eraser only if it is held by some device.

1. Those who cannot hold an eraser alone may manage to use one if it is secured in a large bulldog clip. The bulldog clip will provide a larger, firmer area to grip than the eraser alone (Figure 6.2).
2. It is also possible to make a holder for an eraser using thermoplastic splinting material which is malleable after immersing in hot water (Figure 6.3).
3. Two part epoxy compounds which may be moulded onto the eraser to the required shape may also be used. The size of the grip may be increased as well as the shape which may be modelled according to most effective type of grip of the user. A

Figure 6.3: An eraser held in a thermoplastic grip. The grip may be shaped in various ways so that it suits the type of grip the user is able to adopt.

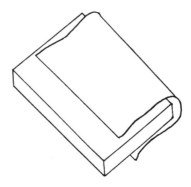

compound should be chosen which will harden at room temperature and does not require heating in an oven; many erasers are made of material which would melt if heated.

4. Pencils may be purchased which have an eraser attached to the non-writing end. Such pencils will provide a suitable grip by which some people may use an eraser. However these erasers are usually small and so have a limited life.

5. Novelty erasers are available which may be fitted over the end of an ordinary pencil or piece of wood dowel.

METHODS OF APPLYING PAINT

For the people who are unable to grade the amount of pressure exerted on the paper a brush is often not the best method of applying paint. The bristles of brushes are pliable so heavy pressure will cause the metal collar which secures the bristles to be in contact with the paper. There are, however, other means of applying paint, some of which may be adapted to suit the needs of an individual.

1. The simplest method of applying paint is with the fingers, the heel or side of the hand, or even the whole hand. This method may be effective for people who are unable to sustain a grip on any kind of tool in the hand. It may be used to encourage fine finger movements, whole hand, arm or body movement depending on the nature of the project undertaken. The shape of the part

of the hand being used will dictate the shape of the paint mark produced and could provide inspiration for design. This makes it a good medium for those lacking confidence in their artistic ability.

It may be undertaken using paint produced specifically as a finger painting medium or made from powder paint bound with starch or paste. Acrylic medium or synthetic resin may also be added to the paint.

Painting may be on paper or on a smooth, washable, non-porous surface, such as a plastic worktop. One or more prints on paper may be made from paintings completed on a smooth surface. Guy Scott describes these techniques in detail in his book, *Introducing Finger Painting* (Scott, 1973). He also describes various other techniques related to finger painting, creating textures with rag, corrugated card, combs etc. in paint which has been applied with the hands.

2. A finger stall with which to apply paint may be fashioned from a piece of plastic foam in which a slit of suitable size is cut to accommodate the finger. This method may be used therapeutically to encourage individual finger movement.

3. To cover a large area with paint a block of plastic foam may be used, held with a whole hand grip. Should such a grip not be possible, a slit through the foam through which tape is threaded which may then be used to secure the foam by tying it round the hand. Alternatively a slit in the block of foam may be used to accommodate the hand.

4. Short-haired brushes may be adapted by shortening the handle and attaching a T-bar for use by people who can only adopt a whole hand horizontal grip (Figure 5.10).

5. For people whose only effective grip is a whole hand vertical one, a foam-tipped painting stick may be effective. This is made from a piece of dowel of a diameter comfortable for the user, with a plastic foam painting tip. The foam may either be a cylinder of high density foam attached to the stick with waterproof glue or a circle cut from a sheet of foam which is then tied over the end of the stick. (See Figure 5.10 for methods of attaching plastic foam to the painting tip.)

6. For people who can adopt a horizontal grip more easily than a vertical or tripod one, a T-shaped painting stick may be suitable. The stick is made from two pieces of dowel attached to each other in a T-shape. Foam is attached to the vertical bar of the T (Figure 5.10).

7. Many home decorators find that using a roller is a quick and efficient method of applying paint. A small version of this type of roller may be used to apply paint to paper. It may be made by adapting a roller intended to seal the seams of wallpaper. The roller should be covered with a thin layer of plastic foam. One roller will be needed for each colour of paint being used during a particular session; thorough washing of a single roller when each type or a different colour of paint is required would be tedious and defeat the aim of having a quick and efficient means of applying paint.

This method of applying paint could be used therapeutically if large sheets of paper are used so that flexion and extension of the elbow is encouraged during vertical strokes and adduction and abduction of the shoulder during horizontal ones.

RULERS

A number of techniques may be used to enable a ruler to be handled more easily.

1. The underside of the ruler may be given an even coat of rubber solution to provide it with a non-slip surface. This technique will obscure slightly the measuration on translucent plastic rulers. It will also raise the surface of the ruler very slightly from the paper which could be a disadvantage where absolute accuracy is required.
2. A strip of plastic non-slip material such as Dycem may be stuck to the underside of the ruler. This material is available in rolls and may be cut with scissors to the exact size required. Again this raises the surface of the ruler from the paper and may reduce accuracy. The measuration on the ruler may also be slightly obscured on translucent plastic rulers though less with lighter coloured non-slip plastic than a darker one.
3. This non-slip plastic material is also available in the form of self adhesive spots, 15 mm and 21 mm in diameter. They are most suitable for rigid rulers. If used at each end of pliable rulers, pressure of the fingers in the middle will cause it to bow. In practice, these spots have been found to be more suitable for use by adults than children. Many children seem to be unable to control the desire to remove them.
4. Perhaps the most effective use of this non-slip plastic material is

Figure 6.4: The underside of a ruler with a finger grip into which a folded strip of non-slip material has been slotted. The diagram on the right shows a section cut through the ruler and the positioning of the non-slip material so that when in use it will be in contact with the surface on which the ruler rests but will not impair accuracy when the ruler is used for measuring.

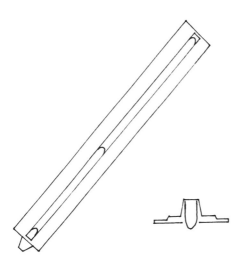

with a ruler which has a raised portion along its centre. On the reverse side this raised portion is hollow and may be filled with a folded strip of non-slip plastic material cut to such a size that it lies flush with the undersurface of the ruler so as not to raise the ruler from the surface of the paper or impair accuracy while measuring (Figure 6.4).

STABILIZING WORK

Most artwork which is applied to paper or other similar material requires that material to be secured by some means.

Securing the base on which the person is working is particularly important for those who have limited hand function or inability to change their position.

Children too will require paper to be secured, even in situations where their peers would work on a piece of paper simply placed on their desk. With the very young child who will spend only a very short time completing a drawing or painting, a method of securing should be chosen that takes little time both to set up and remove.

1. Drawing board clips may be used, of course, on drawing boards but also on any table or desk which has a lip on which the clips will grip.
2. Reusable adhesive putty, such as Blu-tack, is available in a sheet; pieces of the desired size may be pulled off it. Strips of putty are also available, such as Buddies, each of which contain a number of small squares of the putty. The latter may be more suitable for independent use because each piece is of usable size so that it is unnecessary to pull bits from a complete sheet.
3. A non-slip plastic sheet such as Dycem, may be all that is necessary to stabilize the paper from some people. Its suitability will depend on the type of work which is being undertaken, for the plastic does not provide as firm a surface as wood or formica.
4. Drawing pins are only suitable if they do not pose a hazard to the user. The person who is unable to lift their hand from the drawing surface and who must slide it across the surface should not use drawing pins. Repeated use will, of course, damage a drawing board, desk or table top.
5. Self-adhesive Velcro will secure paper, card or other materials when a long term project is being undertaken but would be expensive to use on a regular basis.
6. Double-sided tape may be used if it is not important to be able to remove it completely from the back of the completed piece of work.

The use of the materials described in the preceding pages will enable many people to produce artwork of a standard in keeping with their aspirations. For other people, drawing, painting and technical drawing by the usual means will not be a realistic proposition. For both children and adults, special techniques may be necessary if their output is to enhance self-esteem and motivation, provide a satisfying leisure activity or even a means of augmenting income.

STENCILS AND TEMPLATES

A stencil is made from a sheet of material, card, plastic, wood or

Figure 6.5: a) Simple stencils of basic geometric shapes. b) Thick card stencils of simple objects to encourage children to persist with colouring and ensure an acceptable result.

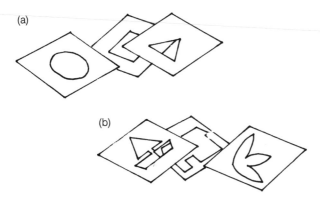

(a)

(b)

metal, from the centre of which the desired shape has been cut. The user works within the limits of the stencil. (Figure 6.5). A template is a piece of suitable material around the edges of which the user works. For people with impaired fine motor function it is usually easier to work within a stencil than around as template because the former provides a rigid limit within which the user works.

1. Stencils of basic geometric shapes are commercially available or they may be home-made. Commercially available stencils are sometimes made from transparent plastic material. This material is excellent where accurate placement is desired in relation to other parts of the piece of work. For people with impaired vision, however, they may be difficult to see when placed on paper. Home-made stencils may be fashioned quickly from thick card, or more durable stencils may be made from hardboard. With these materials the stencil will be more easily seen against the paper (Figure 6.5). These basic stencils are very useful for children who have motor planning difficulties and are delayed in their ability to draw such shapes free-hand. Children who have such difficulties are often deterred from practicing their drawing skills because they are disappointed with their results. The less practice they have the less likely are these skills to improve. Using a stencil under supervision these children achieve good results which motivates further practice. Basic stencils also help the development of motor planning. The child who is not able to draw a

round enclosed shape, organize the precise change of direction necessary to draw a square, or draw the diagonal lines of a triangle, is not aware of how these movements feel. Stencils guide the hand movements, thus providing experience of the sensation of drawing specific shapes and helping to establish motor planning. It is often found that after producing a number of any one shape the memory of the motor plan persists for a while and free-hand shapes may be drawn. Sessions using stencils should be continued until the shape has been learned and may be drawn free-hand at will.

2. Thick card stencils of houses, transport vehicles and the like are helpful for children who have difficulty with fine motor skills. They may be used to encourage the reluctant child to persist with scribbling because the end result will be a recognizable representation of an object. They may also be used whilst encouraging the use of an appropriate pencil grip (Figure 6.5).

3. Smaller stencils stamped out on waxed card may be used by both children and adults. There are usually a number of stencils on one card on a single theme, flowers, farm animals, birds etc. They may be used in a number of ways.

   (a) Using a stencil brush and paint they may be completely filled in with one colour of paint.

   (b) They may be used as an aid to drawing by those who are not sure how to portray a particular object on paper or lack the confidence to make an attempt.

   (c) Novelty effects may be created by drawing round the edge of the stencil with a felt-tipped pen, moving the stencil slightly and repeating the process with a different coloured pen.

   (d) This type of stencil is effective used for the main objects in a picture, the desired background having been previously completed.

   (e) There is a return of the vogue for stencilled furniture and furnishings. A variety of stencils are commercially available which are suitable for use on small articles such as wastepaper bins and kitchen utensils, as well as larger ones intended for use on furniture. Books are available which describe the process in detail (Janitch, 1975; Parry, 1977).

4. Templates, perhaps secured to paper with a small piece of reusable adhesive putty, may be used to achieve novelty effects which do not rely on accurate drawing.

   (a) The template may be outlined with pastel crayon or coloured chalk which is then smudged to create a gradually fading effect. This technique is particularly effective when used for repeating patterns on a paper of contrasting colour.

(b) Templates may also be used to mask parts of the paper, the remainder being coloured with paint or crayon. The resulting picture will have a silhouette effect.

RUBBING

Church brasses have formed the basis of beautiful rubbings for many years. This technique has been so popular in some parts that churches have needed to limit the number of times a brass may be rubbed lest it be rubbed away. Brass rubbing, using heel ball, a shoemakers' polishing mixture of beeswax, tallow and lamp-black or thick wax crayons in the usual range or metallic colours, allows people with little artistic ability or lack of precise motor control to produce interesting designs and decorations. A paper or card frame will obscure any inaccuracy caused by poor motor control.

Rubbings need not be confined to church brasses. Interesting effects may be obtained by rubbing other surfaces (Figure 6.6).

1. The trunks of trees which have interesting bark textures may be rubbed.
2. In some areas it is still possible to find Victorian cast iron covers to coal cellars. Their raised patterns provide the basis for unusual rubbings.
3. Many households will contain furniture with areas of carving or metal objects with designs in relief. So long as it is possible to secure paper over the design it will be possible to make a rubbing.
4. There are many household objects which have interesting textures. Unfinished or heavily weathered pieces of hardwood often have raised grains and knots which will make detailed rubbings.
5. Leaves and ferns arranged with the veined side uppermost make interesting rubbings either used singly or arranged in a pleasing composition.
6. All over patterns may be created by rubbing frosted glass, wire mesh or textured textiles.
7. Objects which children use for rubbing should be small and quickly completed. Coins are ideal because their effect is almost immediate. They may be used for the child who is reluctant to

Figure 6.6: Rubbings with wax crayon. a) From a cut glass dish. b) From a Victorian cast iron fender. c) From ivy leaves.

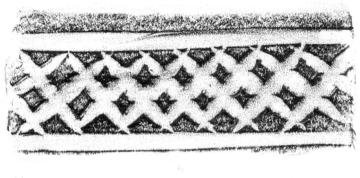

(a)

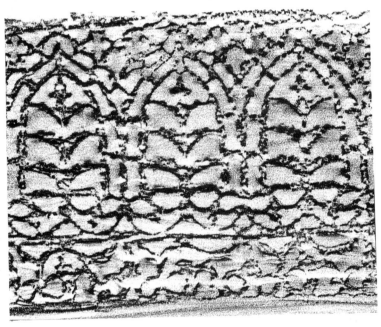

(b)

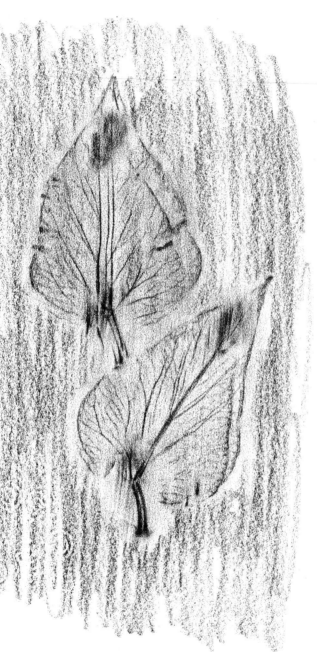

(c)

put crayon to paper because of fear of failure. The desire to see the design appear encourages hand/eye coordination.

SIMPLE TECHNIQUES USING WAX CRAYONS

1. Grated wax crayon may be used to create designs. It can be applied with a brush, if this is possible, or dispensed from a shaker made from a discarded washing-up liquid bottle or similar container. The crayon will, of course, have to be grated to a suitable fineness to pass easily through the nozzle of the container. The sprinkled design may then be amended with the hand, a spatula or piece of card before a piece of sugar (construction) paper is placed over it and a moderately hot iron applied to melt the was and fix it to the paper. The two sheets of paper must be separated before the wax resets.
2. Thick wax crayons may be notched at intervals down their length, thus providing a serrated surface. Held horizontally such crayons will produce several lines of colour at any one time. They are particularly effective for creating twisting or swirling patterns in one or more colours. If necessary it is possible to use a bulldog clip on the crayon to provide a larger area to grip.
3. Wax crayons may be used to achieve many interesting effects. They may be used alone or combined with paint or inks. Some of these techniques could be used by those with motor disabilities. Henry Pluckrose describes many of these techniques in his book, *Introducing Crayon Techniques* (Pluckrose, 1967).

PRINTING

1. Perhaps the simplest method of creating an imprint is with a thumb, finger, hand or even a foot. Single prints are interesting when they are made for the first time perhaps by someone who has never applied paint to a surface before. However, more interesting designs can be made by repetition in either a random or regular fashion.
2. Most people during their school days have carved a design on the cut surface of a potato, applied powder paint and made prints. The potato is a very suitable medium for printing for those who have difficulty with grip, for the part of the potato which is held

in order to make the print may also be carved to produce a shape easily held by the user.

3. Many household objects may be used for printing, either as they are or with the addition of a suitable handle. The tops from bottles which have held soft drinks or cosmetics have patterns embossed on them, as do the rubber ferrules of walking sticks and crutches. Pieces of kitchen equipment, such as potato mashers, graters, balloon egg whisks and pastry cutters, may also be used.

4. Rubber stamps for printing are commercially available. They may be of geometric shapes or objects such as fruits, birds or animals. These may be used simply to print the object depicted upon them or the simpler shapes may be used to embellish pictures and designs. For example, children with limited hand function may enjoy adding leaves with an ellipse shaped stamp to the bare branches of a tree which has been drawn for them. Similarly animal prints may be used to add livestock to a bare farmyard or flowers may be printed onto paper on which there are already flower stems.

MICROCOMPUTERS

The advent of the microcomputer has enlarged the world of art and technical drawing both for people with normal motor abilities and for those with disabilities. For the latter, depression of keys can replace the complex motor manoeuvres of using pencils and geometric instruments. For those unable to use a conventional keyboard, other devices are commercially available or may be custom-made to suit particular needs (Chapter 8).

For professionals and enthusiastic amateurs, graphics may be produced using computer language. These processes are described in the manual which is provided with each microcomputer. Designs may be printed on a dot matrix or ink jet printer; a daisy wheel printer is not suitable for printing graphics. The prints, of course, will be in black and white, the colours which are displayed on the VDU will be depicted on the print as various densities of dots. Colour printers are available, but at present they are too costly to be considered by all but serious microcomputer graphic artists.

A variety of simple graphic programs are commercially available which do not rely on the ability to use the programming language of the microcomputer. These allow the user, having become conversant with the commands used in the program, to 'draw' geometric designs and simple pictures.

So called 'art' programs are available which allow the user to exercise artistic ability to a greater or lesser extent. The simplest of these allow the user to select an object to 'draw' and 'colour' from a limited menu. Such programs are often designed to encourage hand/eye coordination, and teach cause and effect by demonstrating that the sustained depression of a key or special switch produces a result on the VDU.

Other programs provide a pre-selected picture and a choice of colours in which it may be completed. Often the colours are numbered and the colour chosen by depressing the appropriate number on the keyboard.

More complex programs allow the user to draw a picture or design and colour it from a 'palette' which is usually displayed at the side of the VDU screen. This type of programme gives the greater degree of personal choice but the wide range of choices available makes some programs tedious to operate, requiring the cursor to be located on the colour required and then moved to the area where that colour is to be used. Should this, however, be the only realistic means of producing artwork and the user is well motivated the repetitive procedures will be worthwhile.

New art programs are frequently developed both commercially and by amateur enthusiasts. The most fruitful and up-to-date source of information is the large range of magazines published for microcomputer users. Because these are usually published monthly, information of new developments is more recent than that obtainable from books. (See Chapter 8 for further details regarding microcomputers.)

7

Typewriters and electronic printers: teaching keyboard skills

> . . . but Tom had never typed a word in his
> life. Besides, he could neither read nor
> write. With the same quiet determination
> that has characterised each stage of this
> work, Tom taught himself to type laboriously,
> letter by letter, using one finger of each
> hand.
>
> Joseph Deacon, *Tongue Tied*

Typewriters, machines which produce printed words on paper, can help many people who have motor disabilities to record on paper. An unadapted machine may be all that some people need to be able to record effectively on paper, others will need adapted machines and special devices. As far as children are concerned, where there is doubt about a child's ability to write there is nothing to be lost by teaching keyboard skills even if in the future acceptable handwriting skills develop. The child who is delayed in developing handwriting skills has less early practice in sequencing words and sentences on paper and constructing the written word. For the child who is unlikely to develop the skills required for handwriting, a keyboard should be introduced as early as possible. 'It is wasteful and frustrating to child and teacher alike to urge the child to try to write when the task is well nigh impossible' (Bowley, 1969).

A similar statement could be made of adults whose hand function is limited. Adults need to be able to sign their names, but beyond that most other recording and communicating on paper may be accomplished by other means. The content of words on paper is more important than the means by which those words are recorded. Handwriting which is accomplished only with great conscious effort will detract from the amount of concentration and effort which is free to be expended on the content of the work (Figure 7.1).

Figure 7.1: These examples of the handwriting and the first attempt at typewriting of a 14 year old boy who has severe coordination difficulties which were produced on the same day. Typewriting removed the need for complex motor planning and there was an immediate improvement in the content of his work. For the past six months he has attended keyboard classes each Saturday morning and is now using an electric typewriter in school. Not only has the amount of work he is able to produce increased but it is also legible and well presented. He has gained self-confidence and self esteem.

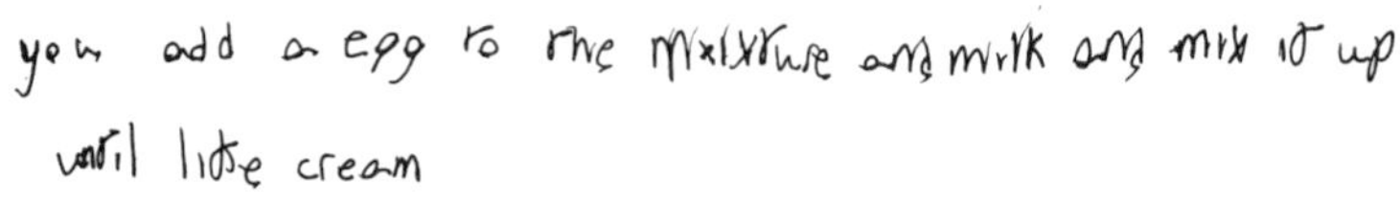

you add a egg to the mixture and mirlk and mix it up
until lile cream

As an object increases in size it gets
bigger than the surface area to the
volume status decreases. i.e. the
surface does not increase.

SYMPTOMS WHICH OCCUR IN BOTH CHILDREN AND ADULTS WHICH SUGGEST THAT TYPEWRITING MAY BE A USEFUL SKILL TO DEVELOP

Motor control difficulties

Typewriters are appropriate for some people who do not have, for a number of reasons, sufficient fine motor control to undertake any writing with a hand held tool.

The reason for this may be caused by difficulty sustaining the grip on a pen or pencil because of limitation of joint movement, lack of power, pain or discomfort.

Neurological impairment may prevent the execution of the movements necessary to form letter characters. Such impairments may be caused by visuo-perceptual difficulties, motor or motor planning deficits.

Alan is 26 years old and has just begun studying for a PhD degree in social studies. He suffers from athetoid cerebral palsy. His first nine years of education were completed without him ever having committed a word to paper, except for this first name, which with great effort and concentration he was able to write in block capitals. Had his name contained any letters with curves in them it is doubtful if he would even have been able to write those few letters.

It was unfortunate that not until the age of 14 was it suggested to him that a keyboard would be appropriate. At this time small electronic printers had just appeared on the market. One of these machines revolutionized Alan's academic career. He was able to use an unadapted machine, steadying his hand on its front edge. After a short time he was proficient enough to use the machine for his school work. It must be remembered that this was the first time Alan had had the means to record on paper and it took time for him to learn to construct written sentences, a skill that his classmates had been practising for nine years.

He was successful in his GCE O'level examinations at the age of 18 and gained sufficient A'levels to be accepted for a degree course at university two years later. When his studies are completed Alan plans to have a career in social work with particular interest in the needs of people with disabilities.

Had not Alan been introduced to a keyboard his academic abilities would never have been manifested. Clearly this is the only way in which he will ever be able to record effectively on paper.

Joint deformity

Joint deformity which occurs in arthritis and arthrogryposis may preclude handwriting because of the unsuitable fixed position of the hand. For those able to accomplish a little handwriting, lack of speed may make it an uneconomic means of recording on paper.

Typing may be more comfortable than handwriting for those people who suffer from joint inflammation or erosion which occurs in rheumatoid or osteo-arthritis. Typing does not require the hand to sustain a grip on a tool, there is gentle finger movement and the appearance of the completed piece of work does not depend on rhythmic sustained movement.

Slow handwriting

The handwriting of some people lacks speed, which may be caused by minimal motor dysfunction or dyspraxia. Writing legibly at speed is important when writing examination papers. At GCSE level a writing speed of between 16 and 20 words per minute is necessary if sufficient information is to be recorded (Chasty, 1986). A typewriter may be a more realistic method of attaining these speeds.

Amy, who suffers from congenital left hemiplegia, is 16 years old and shortly will be writing her first public examination papers. She is a girl with great determination, application and higher than average academic ability. She was referred for advice from an occupational therapist because her handwriting lacked the necessary speed to write examination papers successfully.

Assessment showed that she had a number of problems. As with many people who suffer from congenital hemiplegia, she had slight motor impairment on the right side. In addition, motor effort of the right hand caused spasm in the left which became uncomfortable when undertaking prolonged periods of handwriting. Being an extremely conscientious girl, Amy perseveres for long periods and produces similar amounts of written work to her peers.

Strategies to provide immediate help include holding an object in her left hand whilst handwriting to help to prevent spasm of effort. Learning economy of words so that the maximum information is recorded using the minimum of words. A letter has been written to her examination board with medical and paramedical endorsement requesting extra time to complete examination papers. It is hoped that this extra time will enable her to record sufficient material to gain good grades as well as help her to have a more relaxed attitude during her examinations.

In the longer term Amy has been strongly advised to begin to learn to use a keyboard after her examinations are completed during the three months before she begins her advanced examination course. Thus she should have keyboard skills of at least 20 words per minute in time for her next important written examinations. It is not being suggested that she abandons handwriting but that she types long pieces of written work so that she may adequately demonstrate her abilities.

USE OF TYPEWRITERS AND PRINTERS

Typewriters and electronic printers are helpful for people in many and various situations.

1. Both for people who are unable to undertake any handwriting and those who lack speed and legibility, a keyboard will be appropriate for recording on paper in school and further education.
2. Keyboard skills may be necessary at work. Typing may be the chosen career or acquired disability may make a change of occupation to one which includes typing necessary.
3. Typing may be the only means by which a person may pursue an interest in creative writing of articles, stories or poems.
4. Other interests and hobbies require words to be recorded on paper. A typewriter may be the best means of continuing correspondence with penfriends. Housebound people may be able to help with the preparation of paperwork for community projects by means of a typewriter, this not only fulfilling a useful role but also increasing their contact with their local community.

THE FACILITIES PROVIDED BY VARIOUS KINDS OF TYPEWRITERS AND ELECTRONIC PRINTERS

Typewriters may be mechanical, known as manual machines, have keys which are electrically fired, or be sophisticated machines which have an electronic display which allows the text to be viewed and, if necessary, corrected before it is printed. Some machines have a memory which allows text to be saved, edited or rearranged.

In order to make an appropriate choice to suit the abilities and disabilities of a particular user the qualities of each type of machine must be considered.

Manual typewriters

These may be full-size office models which are robust and intended for prolonged use or portable ones intended for occasional domestic use. The former are heavy and not easily portable. They need to be set up in a position in which they will be used and covered when not in use to prevent dust collecting on and in them. Those requiring such a machine will need to buy a second hand machine as they are no longer manufactured today.

Although small manual machines are described as 'portable' many of them weigh too much to be easily carried for more than short distances. Most portable manual typewriters have their own carrying case which gives them a neat appearance and make them easily portable within the home or by car. These machines are made for home use and not intended to be used for many hours each and every day. These machines are still manufactured and are comparatively inexpensive to buy.

Advantages of manual typewriters

1. They are inexpensive to buy.
2. Being mechanical they do not need to be used where an electric outlet is available.

Disadvantages of manual typewriters

1. Parts necessary to repair an office model will be difficult to obtain.
2. The keys need to be struck very sharply in order that the print is clear. The imprint of the characters on the paper depends entirely on the manner in which the key is struck, thus an inconsistent strike will produce irregular printed characters. Unlike electric typewriters, which usually have square keys, manual typewriters keys are often round and this, combined with the comparatively steep slope at which the rows of keys are set means that there is a considerable space between the keys which can be a hazard when used by people with less than perfect motor control. The impact of a finger thrust between the keys can be very painful. Such machines are rarely suitable for people who have any type of hand disability, whether it be neurological, articular or lack of power.
3. The carriage return is operated by a lever which requires the hand to be lifted above the keyboard to the left of the machine and moved towards the right.
4. Ribbons for manual machines are on spools. The ribbon needs to be handled in order to thread it through the clips in front of the platen and on to the spool at the other side of the machine. This not only means that the hands will be soiled but also that the person with the impaired hand function may need help with fitting a new ribbon.

5. With some machines the ribbon needs to be rewound in order to reuse it. There is a small crank with handle provided for this purpose but rewinding requires dexterity and sustained movement.

6. Care should be taken when choosing a portable machine, for some models have a short platen which will only take A4 paper inserted vertically. A4 paper may not be used horizontally nor may a larger size of paper be used. Few of them will accept the thickness of a substantial A4 envelope.

Electric typewriters.

Portable models may still be purchased but the large office model has been superseded by electronic machines and word processors. Office models may be purchased second hand but it is becoming more difficult to obtain the spare parts which may be required to repair machines.

Advantages of electric typewriters

1. The characters produced on the paper are consistently clear because the imprinting of them depends on the electric firing of the key, not on the type and strength of the strike of the user on the keys. They are thus suitable for a user who has fluctuating muscle power, lack of power or limitation of movement.
2. The carriage return is usually operated by one of the keys on the keyboard so that no more movement is required than to activate other functions of the machine.
3. Similarly, the paper feed is usually operated by a single key. The user, therefore does not require a reciprocal pronation/supination movement to insert or remove paper.

Disadvantages of electric typewriters

1. They may only be used where an electric outlet is available. This will be particularly relevant in schools, where it may be found that the position of the electric outlet means that the child must sit apart from his peer group or in a position which makes it difficult to participate fully in classroom activities such as being able to see what is written on a chalkboard. (In many classrooms the electric socket is under the chalkboard.) The difficulties may

become more urgent when a child begins secondary eduction and each subject is taught in a different room and a new power point must be located perhaps seven or more times each day.

2. The so called 'portable' models are indeed portable but many of them weigh as much as 5 kg, which begins to feel very heavy when they are carried frequently or for more than a few metres.

Electronic typewriters

There is a great variety of electronic machines which may be purchased today. They vary greatly in their degree of sophistication and the number of functions they are capable of. Careful thought should be given to the functions which are required or may be required in the future. It is futile to pay for features which never will be used. In addition, a large number of keys which have symbols which are not understood can be confusing to the user. This is particularly true when the symbols of more than one function are depicted on a single key.

Some features of electronic typewriters

1. They are much quieter in use than manual and electric typewriters. This is important in a classroom and other situations where noise may disturb other people.
2. Some machines have the option of mains or battery power supply; batteries may be of the rechargeable variety. Battery power, of course, frees the user from the need of an electric outlet so that the machine may be used in whatever situation it is needed. This is particularly useful for children of secondary school age who move between several classrooms during their school day and who need to use a keyboard for most of their recording on paper.
3. Ribbons are housed in cassettes making them clean and easy to insert. The ribbon is not exposed so the hands do not touch it. The cassette is usually fitted by pressing it into position, making it easy to insert by a person with a minimum of finger movement.

    Several types of ribbon are available. The types available for a particular machine should be ascertained before purchase.

    (a) Fabric ribbon is the most economical to use because it is automatically rewound within the cassette. Its usage is limited only by fading of the print which of course occurs as the amount of ink remaining on the ribbon decreases. The print from a fabric ribbon is initially good but it is never as sharp as that of a carbon ribbon.

(b) Carbon film ribbon may either single or multi-strike. The single strike film moves so that each letter character strikes an unused part of the ribbon. A multi-strike film moves more slowly so that the ribbon moves only fractionally for each letter character that is struck, the successive character overlapping the area which was used by the previous one. Both of these types of ribbon are used only once after which a new cassette must be inserted. These ribbons usually cost slightly less than reusable fabric ribbons but because of their once only use the overall cost is greater. Single and multi-strike carbon ribbons provide a very sharp, professional looking print, the single strike being slightly superior.

4. Many electronic typewriters print letter characters by means of a daisy wheel. This is a disc which has a number of spokes arranged round the perimeter, one for each character which may be printed. When a key is struck the daisy wheel spins until the appropriate character is in the exact position to be printed. Daisy wheels are usually contained within a cassette and are easy to remove and insert. Daisy wheels of various print styles may be obtained.

5. Only a light finger touch is required to fire the keys of an electronic typewriter. This is an advantage for people who lack power in the fingers. For other people the delicate touch which is required could be a disadvantage. This would be so for people who have difficulty initiating movement and releasing pressure because many machines have keys which automatically repeat if pressure is sustained. It is advisable to look at and test the reaction of keys to pressure before a purchase is made.

6. Some machines have an illuminated display of characters so that corrections and alterations may be made before the characters are printed. The size of the display varies between models. Care should be taken when choosing a model which has an illuminated display because the visibility varies between models. The characters are usually depicted by a series of dots or lines, similar to those on a pocket calculator. The colour of the display is also significant, particularly for those with visual deficit; some colours may be seen more easily than others. The contrast between the background colour and that of the characters may not be sufficient for some people with poor vision. The angle at

Figure 7.2: Right justification.

```
Some machines have a facility which
allows the right margin to be justified;
the right margin will be straight in the
same way as the left one. This is a
useful facility for people who wish to
produce pamphlets, booklets newsletters
etc. because the page will look rather
like a printed one.
```

which the display window is set in the facia of the machine is also important. People with limited head or trunk movement may not be able to adjust their position in order to see the display clearly.

7. Some machines have a facility which allows the right margin to be justified; the right margin will be straight in the same way as the left one is (Figure 7.2). This is useful for people who wish to produce pamphlets, booklets, newsletters etc. because the page will look rather like a printed one. However justification of the right margin is not recommended for letters or typescripts for publishing because in the first instance it is said that right justification is more difficult to read in letter form. In the second instance right justification makes estimating wordage difficult.

8. A conventional typewriter allocates exactly the same amount of space to each letter character. Some characters occupy more space than others, for example i fills less space than w. On a typewritten page there will therefore be more space between some characters than others. Some electronic typewriters have a facility which allows the letters to be spaced proportionally, that is as they are on the printed page where less space is allocated to some characters than others so that the space between characters is more or less equal. The resultant page looks almost like a printed one (Figure 7.3).

9. Some models have a facility which allows paper to be fed automatically into a machine. These may be normal cut sheets of paper such as A4, or fan folded paper by means of a tractor feed. These are usually optional additions to the basic machine. Their cost is quite substantial but would be justified if they enabled a person to use the typewriter independently.

Figure 7.3: Proportional spacing.

A conventional typewriter allocates exactly the same amount of space to each letter character. Some characters occupy more space than others, for example 'i' fills less space than 'w'. On a typewritten page there will, therefore, be more space between some characters than others. Some electronic typewriters have a facility which allows the letters to be spaced proportionally as in this example.

Electronic printers

There are machines which are not strictly speaking typewriters, which electronically allow the user to produce words on paper. The print produced by them is similar to that of a dot matrix printer in that characters are formed by a number of dots. The larger the number of dots present in each printed character the clearer it appears. The dots which form the characters are burned onto the paper.

Advantages of electronic printers

1. Some of these machines are very small and lightweight. Some weigh as little as 2.5 kg, which makes them truly portable and particularly suitable for students who must move between different areas of a school or college.
2. They are mains or battery powered, which gives the user freedom of use in any situation.
3. The dimensions of some models are as small as a piece of A4 paper, which means that they may be used at a small desk or work station and still leave sufficient space for reference books and papers.
4. In addition to printing letter characters some of these machines may also be used to print graphs and diagrams which are useful facilities for students.
5. They cause little disturbance to other people as they emit very little noise.

Disadvantages of electronic printers

1. Because the formation of print requires heat, either special thermal paper or special ribbon is required which is relatively expensive particularly if large quantities are needed.

2. The size of paper which may be used is governed by the size of the platen and the size of the thermal paper which is available.
3. It is not usually possible to make carbon copies. Further copies must be obtained by photocopying.
4. Because of the method of printing, the print appears low down on the platen which makes the line of characters which is currently being printed difficult to read.
5. They are fairly delicate and though they would fit inside a school bag or satchel they will not withstand the rough handling which they may receive in the hand of young children and their friends.

ADAPTATIONS FOR USE WITH TYPEWRITERS AND ELECTRONIC PRINTERS

Keyguards

These are devices which fit over a keyboard and help the user to fire the desired key. Keyguards have an aperture above each of the keys of the keyboard. The keyguard is positioned so that it lies a few millimetres above the keys (Figure 7.4). The user of the keyboard must insert a finger into the appropriate hole in the keyguard in order to fire the key. In this way the person who has tremor, athetosis or other disorder of movement is enabled to use a keyboard more accurately.

The keyguard also provides a base on which the hand may rest while typing which also helps provide stability for the hand which exhibits involuntary movement.

A further use of a keyguard is with children who are beginning to use a keyboard. Sometimes it is desirable to expose only a small number of the keys in the early stages of learning to use the keyboard, either because a young child would be confused by a large array of keys or because an older child has difficulty with figure/background discrimination. The keyguard allows keys to be covered or revealed as desired by temporarily covering parts of the guard with paper or card.

Keyguards may be made of metal or plastic. They may be attached to the keyboard permanently by drilling the outer casing of the keyboard and securing with screws, washers and nuts. Should the guard be a temporary measure it may be attached to the keyboard by means of double-sided adhesive pads. Alternatively the keyguard may be

Figure 7.4: Two types of keyboard. a) A keyboard which is fixed above the keyboard with screws which pass through holes drilled in the fascia of the keyboard. b) A keyguard which fits over the keyboard enclosing the top and sides of it.

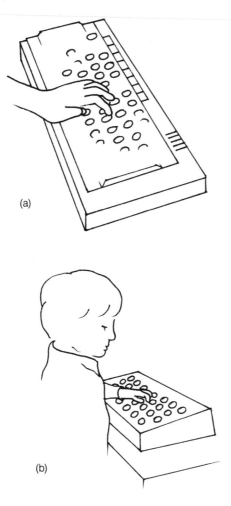

(a)

(b)

constructed with clips which will grip the sides of the keyboard.

Keyguards to suit some keyboards are manufactured commercially. It is possible to make keyguards for specific keyboards for which commercial versions are not available. The position of the apertures must be calculated very accurately so that they are aligned exactly above each key. The apertures are most easily cut in metal using a

Figure 7.5: A typewriter tilted towards the operator by placing it on a wedge.

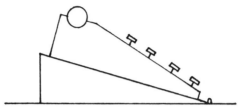

die of appropriate size. Care must be taken to ensure that no rough edges or sharpness is left on the edges of the apertures which could damage the fingers. This is very important for all users, but particularly so for those who do not have precise finger movement and are therefore more likely to bring their fingers in contact with the edges of the apertures.

Arm rests

These help people who are able to use their fingers on the keyboard, but are unable to maintain the hands or arms in an appropriate position. Arm rests may be made from wood, plastic or metal; they may be a flat strip of suitable proportions or shaped to accommodate the forearm. The rest should extend from the front of the keyboard and be long enough to support the whole of the forearm in such a position that the wrists may be held in a mid or slightly extended position. They may be attached to the work surface which accommodates the keyboard by means of a G-clamp or other device.

Arm rests help to give stability for the person who suffers from involuntary movement. They also give support where there is lack of muscle power in conditions such as muscular dystrophy. They provide support and joint protection in painful conditions such as rheumatoid arthritis.

Wedges

A wedge on which a typewriter rests will be useful for those who find extreme downward gaze uncomfortable. It raises the level of the platen which supports the paper as letter characters are imprinted on it, which makes it easier to see what has just been typed. The tilted position in which the typewriter is held encourages the typist to look forward rather than down, thus improving the posture of the neck and shoulders (Figure 7.5).

Tony is a bright, nine-year-old, junior school boy. He suffers from peroneal muscle atrophy which results in progressive muscle weakness, particularly of the distal parts of his limbs. During his early days in the infant department of his school be managed to use a pencil reasonably well. Gradually it became more difficult for him to control a pencil though the small amount of writing he did produce was, and still is, even and legible.

Whilst Tony was still able to write quite easily, an electric typewriter was introduced and a teacher who was experienced in teaching children with disabilities as well as teaching typewriting regularly came into his school to instruct him in keyboard skills. As a result of learning these skills, he has regained his enthusiasm for recording on paper and has developed an interest in writing poetry.

Tony's disability is progressing at a more rapid rate than was earlier anticipated so that his sitting position whilst typing has had to be carefully re-assessed. He sits on a chair which provides support for his back. In order to remove the need for him to flex his upper spine and thus retain the support which his chair provides for his back, a wedge has been introduced on which his typewriter rests. This raises the position of the platen considerably so that he monitors the material he as just typed by looking forwards and not down. He has also been provided with a rest for his forearms which helps to prevent fatigue in that part.

Tony is making good academic progress. The amount of written work he produces is equal to that of his most able peers. Recently a charitable organization has provided for him a second electric typewriter for home use. An added bonus of learning keyboard skills at this stage is that Tony is more than usually proficient when his class is doing microcomputer work.

Head sticks

For people who have insufficient motor control to use the hands to operate any type of keyboard, a head stick may enable them to do so. This is a stick which is attached to some form of headband or helmet and is suitably angled for the person to be able to fire the appropriate keys with it (Figure 7.6). Various head harnesses have been devised, the choice must be made to suit individual needs. The

Figure 7.6: A head stick attached to a head harness which may be used for firing the keys of an electric or electronic keyboard. Head sticks may also be fitted with a device to hold a pencil or brush.

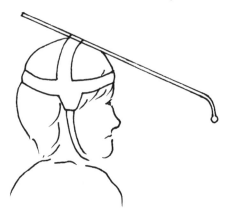

head stick may be attached at the top of the head harness or at forehead level. The latter position probably gives the user more accurate control though the former position is safer. A head stick which is attached to the harness at forehead level is not suitable for people who have involuntary movement, such as occurs in some types of cerebral palsy or dystonia, because of the danger of self injury should the stick be hit against some hard object. The addition of a keyguard over the typewriter keys will help to prevent the user of the head stick from depressing the wrong key.

Hand-held sticks

A hand-held T-stick may aid typing for people who have no individual finger movement but have a stable horizontal whole hand grip. The bar should be fashioned so that it is comfortable to hold according to the needs of the person using it. Slight indentations to accommodate each finger add to the comfort of the grip. Alternatively the grip may be padded with soft foam rubber. The addition of a strap over the back of the hand will prevent the T-stick being dropped by those who cannot sustain a grip for a long period of time. The tip of the stick which is in contact with the keyboard should be of a non-abrasive, non-slip material (Figure 7.7).

For people with only a vertical whole hand grip a simple stick with a non-slip tip may be used.

Figure 7.7: A typing stick with a strap which fits over the back of the hand so that it is not dropped if the grip of it is released.

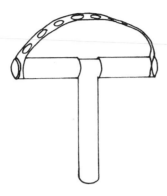

Splints

Some people who do not have voluntary extension of individual fingers may be helped to use those fingers for typing if they are taped in an extended position. Alternatively a small splint made from thermoplastic material may be used. For other people the problem may be the inability to use fingers individually and isolating those which are to be used for typing. Taping the fingers which are not being used in a flexed position against the palm of the hand may be effective.

For some people the best hand function results when the elbows are extended. Elbows may be maintained in extension either by applying gaiters or splints. Where necessary a splint which maintains the arm in extension may incorporate a typing stick for those who also lack the necessary hand function to fire the typewriter keys with the fingers or hold a typing stick.

OTHER TYPES OF KEYBOARD

Expanded keyboards

A larger keyboard than is provided by the typewriter itself may be added to electric and electronic keyboards. The expanded keyboard contains the same range of keys as the keyboard of the typewriter but the keys have a much larger striking area and there is a larger space between one key and the next than on the usual keyboard.

Usually the keys fit flush with the surrounding area of the keyboard until they are depressed, so that even people with very erratic movement are not in danger of trapping their fingers between the keys. The expanded keyboard is electrically connected to the normal typewriter and is usually placed in front of it.

Mini-keyboards

These are small keyboards made for people who have a limited range of movement which would be insufficient to allow them to use a normal sized keyboard. They enable people who suffer from conditions such as muscular dystrophy or osteogenesis imperfecta (brittle bones) to use a keyboard.

Scanning devices

Electric typewriters can also have scanning systems connected to them which are usually controlled by some form of switching device. The characters of the typewriter keyboard are displayed on a screen and are illuminated sequentially. This may proceed row by row and when the row which contains the required character is reached the sequence is stopped. The scanning then continues along that row when the scanning is stopped at the required letter and is then typed. The screen may be controlled by any of a large variety of switches which may be operated by a hand, foot or other part of the body. Such devices enable a typewriter to be used by severely disabled people. However these very specially adapted typewriters are now used much less frequently than in the past. Microcomputers are now used much more frequently because they have a much larger range of functions than simply recording words on paper.

OTHER DEVICES FOR USE IN CONJUNCTION WITH TYPEWRITERS

Lists

People who use typewriters frequently need to be able to refer to various lists. Names and addresses need to be checked and other information referred to. Many young school children use a small

Figure 7.8: A personal telephone directory with press-button operation may be used as a file for people who have difficulty turning the flimsy pages of notebooks.

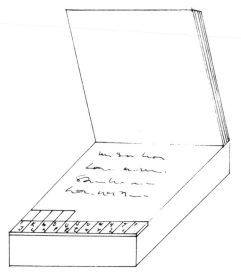

notebook in which they record the spellings of words they have not previously encountered. For people who are unable to handle the small and often flimsy papers of a notebook, a press-button telephone index will provide a means of readily referring to items in alphabetical lists (Figure 7.8).

Page turners

Copy typing sometimes entails turning the pages of a book. A simple page turner consists of a handle with a non-slip plastic blade (Figure 7.9). Another method of making the leaves of a book easier to turn is to slip a paper clip onto the outer edge of each leaf. These will hold the leaves fractionally apart thus making single leaves easier to grip and turn.

Stands

Stands to support material which is being copied are commercially available or may be home-made (Figure 7.10). These stands are

Figure 7.9: A simple page turner with non-slip plastic blade.

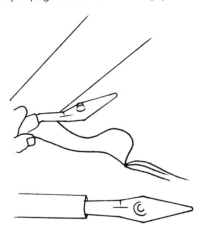

Figure 7.10: A home-made perspex stand for supporting material for reference or copying whilst typing.

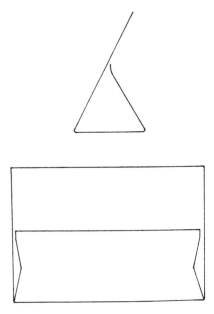

particularly helpful for people who work best with their typewriter supported on a wedge to raise it from the horizontal. A book stand or support will ensure that material which is being copied is at a similar angle to the typewriter.

TEACHING KEYBOARD SKILLS

There are a number of factors to to taken into consideration before deciding the skills which will be necessary for a particular person to employ a keyboard to maximum effect.

1. The purposes for which the keyboard will be used.
2. The nature of motor impairment.
3. The type of keyboard which will be used.
4. Special devices which may be used to activate the keyboard.

Let us consider first, children who will use a keyboard. It will be obvious in the early years of life of some children that they will never have adequate fine motor control to allow them to write with a pen or pencil. Severe cerebral palsy of spastic or athetoid type is an example of such a condition. At the developmental age when children of normal ability are beginning to enjoy making marks on paper, the child with severe motor impairment, should, whenever possible, be given the opportunity to do the same by whatever method is appropriate to the motor impairment which is present.

It is not necessary for the child to have advanced reading skills before he or she is introduced to a keyboard. Pre-school age children may be taught to 'colour' pictures using a typewriter in a similar way to how others would use crayons. At the same time the child will become familiar with the use of a keyboard and how it can be used as a means of self-expression. The position of letter characters on the keyboard will be learned. This is the Goad picture approach to teaching typewriting (Goad, 1977)

Simple outline pictures are prepared of objects with which the child is familiar, three or four objects beginning with each letter of the alphabet (Figure 7.11). Lower case letters clearly written on adhesive paper are superimposed on each key, a different colour of ink being used for the letters of each row. At first all the keys except the one being used are covered with card. An outline picture is inserted in the typewriter and the child is shown how to depress

115

Figure 7.11: Outline pictures for young children to 'colour' using the appropriate letter character so that positions of characters on a keyboard may be learned.

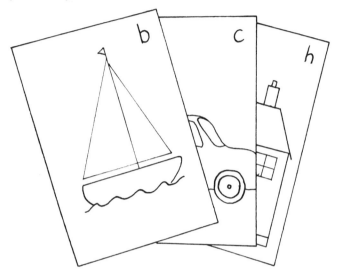

the key, the one with the initial letter of the picture which is being used. The key is fired repeatedly until the picture has been coloured with its initial letter.

Maureen Goad suggests beginning with letters on the middle row of the keyboard, followed by the top row and then the bottom one. She further suggests omitting to teach the letter q until a later stage when it may be taught together with u, which follows it. Omitting q also avoids confusion with the similarly shaped letter p, which is situated at the opposite end of the same row of letters. She suggests that having learned the position of letter characters on the keyboard the child should proceed to learn the use of the space bar and the shift key in order to produce capital letters.

This method of providing a child with basic keyboard skills has also been found to be effective for children who have learning difficulties and do not have the concentration or motivation to work through even a simplified system of learning keyboard skills by conventional methods.

There are other children whose motor disabilities are not so severe as to preclude entirely the use of pens and pencils. These are children who will have enjoyed early attempts at applying paint to

116

paper and scribbling with crayons or felt-tipped pens. Their attempts at drawing specific objects may not have been so successful, and frustration and a disinclination to attempt drawing may have ensued. As schooldays progress these children will probably understand the significance of letter characters and they may appear to write them as successfully as their peers. At the stage when writing has become an unconscious activity for most children, these children will continue to need to concentrate on letter character construction and thus will not be free to give their attention to the content of their written work. Such children will benefit from learning keyboard skills which they may then use for a proportion of their recording on paper.

It has been found that by teaching such children to use a keyboard, providing them with a second method of recording on paper, that there is a spontaneous improvement in their handwriting skills. This may be because the child feels less stressed when a method of recording on paper is provided which does not entail complex motor planning skills. Teaching a child to type indicates that handwriting difficulties have been recognized. A child learning to type must have special individual attention from the teacher of typing. Any or all of these factors may play a part in removing stress, increasing self-esteem and often improving handwriting and the child's attitude towards it.

Not only young children benefit from learning to use a keyboard. Adults whose physical disabilities preclude handwriting may use typing as a means of recording on paper. It is not necessarily those who intend to produce large amounts of work who benefit. Many people who have moderate or severe learning difficulties and will never produce a great deal of work recorded on paper or will never have profound information to record can benefit from learning to use a keyboard. They gain self-esteem and confidence from seeing their own words on paper looking neat and legible. Because recording by means of a typewriter does not require precise or complex motor planning skills, more attention may be given to the content of work which improves in both quality and quantity.

> Laura is an 18-year-old young woman who suffers from moderately severe learning difficulties. She suffers from perceptuo-motor difficulties which have made learning the skills of daily living a very long process. She has both gross and fine motor impairment. She is very much aware of her disabilities which affects her attitudes to tasks which are difficult for her to accomplish.

Handwriting has always been a problem because of motor, motor planning and perceptual problems. Understandably she always has been reluctant to commit words to paper despite having reading skills at a nine to ten year old level. Her school has been reluctant to encourage the use of a typewriter, preferring to persevere with handwriting practice.

Laura, however, does enjoy using an electric typewriter at home which she is far more enthusiastic about than pens and pencils. Using her typewriter she enjoys copying stories from books, copying recipes (she is a keen cook) and constructing short sentences of her own. This is one of the few occupations which she will undertake without her mother's supervision.

Later this year Laura will begin a residential course to improve her independence skills. It is hoped that this course will include a module where she may work to improve her keyboard skills. Laura will not become an accomplished typist but improving her skills will provide a realistic means of recording on paper, an independent activity and a skill which will raise her self-esteem and confidence (Figure 7.12).

Some people will be able to learn to type using a conventional typewriting manual or by attending appropriate classes. Other people have physical, intellectual or perceptual needs which will necessitate special tuition.

A SIMPLIFIED METHOD OF TEACHING KEYBOARD SKILLS

1. Depending on the person's knowledge of the upper and lower case representations of letter characters, the characters on the keys may need to be superimposed with lower case ones.
2. The person is taught to use one finger of the left hand to strike keys which would normally be struck with the left hand and one finger of the right hand for keys which are normally struck with the right hand. It is helpful to colour code the keys to emphasize the hand which must be used, perhaps red for the left hand and green for the right. For the person who has difficulty differentiating between these colours alternatives may be chosen or for the person with little or no colour discrimination a distinctive symbol could be used to indicate the hand to be used.
3. It may not be immediately obvious how many fingers the person will eventually be able to employ effectively when typing. For this reason it is suggested that a vertical method of teaching the

Figure 7.12: An example of Laura's handwriting and typewriting.

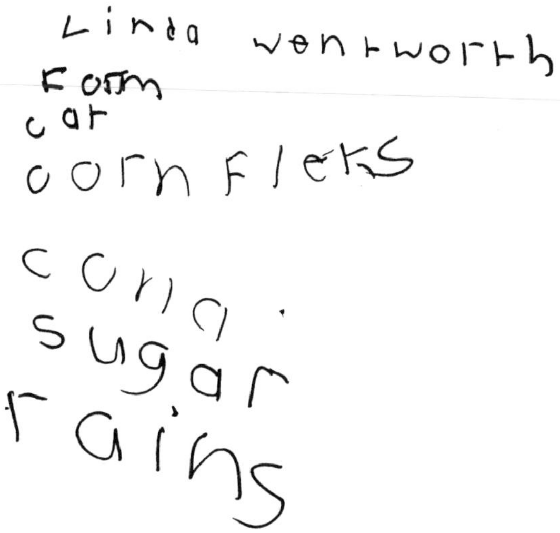

Linda wentworth
form
car
corn fleks

coria .
sugar
rains

I live   at swinton malton york shie

my favourite food is fish and chips

my favour ite drink is reben

My favourite televion program is east ends

10 + 12 = 22

4 + 3 = 8

4 + 3 = 7

keyboard should be used. This applies both to children and adults in whom there may be some doubt as to eventual fingering. The vertical method, while encouraging the correct position of the hands above the keyboard and thus correct fingering, allows some latitude in the number of fingers used.

4. Whatever method of teaching the keyboard is adopted, the home keys, the keys over which the fingers initially lie and always return to, are the same.

   These are:

   (a) Left hand: A, S, D and F.

   (b) Right hand: J, K, L and ; .

   Should it not be possible to use all the fingers the position above the keys to which the fingers always return must be adjusted accordingly. The thumbs are used for the space bar.

5. There is a series of exercises which, when completed, ensure that the position of all the letters characters of the key have been learned. It is important not to perform the exercises only as a mechanical drill but say the letters, either aloud or silently, as each key is struck. Either the name of the letter character or the sound it represents should be used according to the typists usual habit.

Left hand:	Right hand:
fgf (index finger)	jhj (index finger)
frfvf (index finger)	jujmj (index finger)
ftfbf (index finger)	jyjnj (index finger)
dedcd (middle finger)	kik,k (middle finger)
swsxs (ring finger)	lol.l (ring finger)
aqaza (little finger)	;p;/; (little finger)

The characters depicted on the keys used for the last exercise for the right hand may vary on different keyboards. It may be decided not to teach this last exercise in total but only p because the other symbols will not be used frequently.

6. Each exercise should be set out on a separate card which describes exactly what the typist should do together with an example of the completed exercise. Each card should be colour coded or marked with a symbol to indicate which hand the child should use. Each card should also indicate which finger should be used and where spaces should be inserted (Figure 7.13).

7. People who have difficulty with spacing between words when writing should be taught to leave two spaces between words when

Figure 7.13: Keyboard exercises, each on a separate card which are colour coded according to the hand to be used. Each card denotes the finger to be used, exactly what should be typed and an example of the completed exercise.

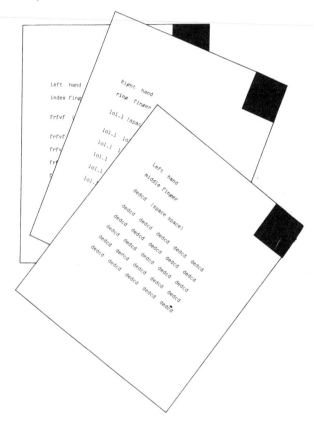

typing. When practising the exercises the spaces should be vocalized as well as the letter names or sounds. Thus the first exercise will be, f-g-f-space (or space-space).

8. The length of each line of typing should be set so that it contains approximately as many characters as the handwriting of that person. In practice this is usually between 30 and 50 characters. Similarly the spaces between lines should be set so that the line width is roughly the same as that between lines of handwriting. Usually double spacing is suitable.

9. When the 12 keys in the centre of the keyboard, those which are ideally struck with the index fingers, have been learned it is

121

possible to form some words. People who already have some word building skills will be able to suggest words which can be made with these letters. This will be the first attempt to use more than one finger within an exercise. Write each word which is to be typed on card, colour coding the letters according to which hand is to be used. In order to prevent the omission of spaces it is advisable that the letters of the word are repeated as it is typed with addition of the space or spaces if more than one space between words is to be taught. Thus 'dog' will be taught as d-o-g-space, 'big' will be typed as b-i-g-space.

At least one complete line of each word should be typed so that the rhythm of the fingering is established. The number of words written on each card will vary according to the abilities of the typist. People who have difficulty with visual fixation will cope better at this stage with only one word on each card. As further keys are learned an increasing variety of words will be possible.

10. Typewriters usually have some auditory signal that the end of a line of type is approaching. This usually occurs six or seven spaces before the end of the line. The typist should learn not to begin a new word or group of letters of an exercise after this signal. At the end of the current word or group of letter characters the carriage return should be struck to return the carriage or print head to the left hand side of the page and move the paper up to the appropriate position for the next line of typing. Whenever possible the carriage return should be struck with the little finger of the right hand. If it is not possible to use the little finger, the finger nearest to the right which can strike this key should be used.

11. Having learned the keyboard and how to type single words the next stage is learning how to produce upper case letter characters in the most efficient way. Except for those who are only able to use one hand for typing the shift lock should not be used for this purpose. The exception would be when a heading is being typed entirely in upper case letter characters. For typing a single upper case letter character the shift key should be depressed with the little finger of the hand which is not being used to type the character. For example, to type upper case G the shift key will be depressed with the little finger of the right hand and the G key with the index finger of the left hand. To type upper case U the shift key will be depressed with the little finger of the left hand and the U key with the index finger of the right hand. The process of typing upper case letter

characters should be: depress the appropriate shift key, press the letter key, release the shift key. Upper case letter may be practised by typing names of family and friends, addresses, days of the week, months, countries, choices depending on the educational level and interest of the child.

12. The next stage is simple copy typing using simple sentences of individual interest. Continue if necessary to colour code the letters according to the hand to be used.

13. It is a big step to progress from copy typing to composing work and typing it. Two devices may be used to help progression to this stage.

    (a) The piece of work to be typed is first dictated by the typist and written down for him or her, still colour coded if necessary. The piece is then copy typed.

    (b) Cards are prepared on which are typed sentences from which one word has been omitted. The typist chooses the word to fill the space. Examples of such sentences may be as simple or as complex as educational and developmental level suggest, for example:

        My name is ——————————.
        My friend is ——————————.
        I like ——————————.
        My birthday is ——————————.

14. To ensure that the paper will be aligned with the rows of print, turn the platen or repeatedly press the carriage return key until 3 or 4 cm of paper is visible. Release the tension on the platen and pull the paper through, aligning the two top corners with the bottom two, return the lever to apply platen tension. Turn the paper down to the required position at the top of the page. For the typist who is unable to insert single sheets of paper, a continuous roll may be used.

15. Learning to type is a tedious process. It is important to demonstrate that the skills which are being learned have practical use, by introducing words which are in the typist's vocabulary as soon as possible. Short frequent practice periods are more effective than longer less frequent ones. Three or four minutes practice every day will soon begin to show results. It is often effective to use a timer for practice periods, finishing the session the second the time limit has expired. This is more conducive to regular practice than prolonging practice until the typist is tired and frustrated.

TYPING WITH ONE HAND OR A LIMITED NUMBER OF FINGERS

There are a number of reasons for a person not being able to use all the fingers for typing.

1. Congenital or acquired deficiency of one or more fingers.
2. Neurological conditions which preclude the use of some fingers, frequently the ring and little fingers, or one hand in conditions such as congenital or acquired hemiplegia.
3. Limitation of finger movement in arthritic and rheumatological conditions.
4. Uncontrolled movement such as tremor and dystonia.
5. Lack of power in conditions such as the muscular atrophies and dystrophies.

Where only a limited number of fingers can be used to type, alternative fingering must be evolved. For the one handed typist the home keys would be F, G, H and J. The fingers placed above these keys would depend, of course, on whether the right or the left hand is being used. From this home position a suitable fingering for the other keys may be planned. Typing manuals are available for one handed typists (Richardson, 1959). Where the typist has a little function in the other hand, though not agile individual finger movement, it may be possible to use that hand to strike the space bar and carriage return and perhaps depress the shift key. This occasional use of the hand with only limited function is desirable in hemiplegia to help maintain a symmetrical position. This is particularly important with children.

One handed typists, depending on the reasons for one handed typing, may attain speeds of 20 or more words a minute.

Faye is 17 years old and suffers from congenital left hemiplegia. She attends her local technical college taking a course in hotel reception work. During her last two years at school she followed a typing course and, though she was only able to use her right hand on the keyboard, attained accurate speeds of 25 words per minute. She hopes that this speed will be sufficient for the amount of typing which will be required of her as a hotel receptionist.

There are other people who will have the use of both hands but not all fingers on each hand, with a little ingenuity it will be possible to devise a system of fingering suitable for most deficits (Crooks, undated).

For people with neurological abnormalities, learning to type will provide problems specific to their particular deficit. For some it may be that exercises intended to teach the keyboard are counter-productive. The effort of typing and the time which elapses between the intent to strike a key and the striking of it allows ample time to locate that key. Some such people will gain maximum proficiency by practising typing words rather than the usual keyboard exercises.

For some people a typewriter may not be of practical use; the word processing element of a microcomputer may provide more potential. The difference in cost between a quality electric typewriter and a word processor is becoming smaller. The additional facilities provided by a microcomputer should be considered. Both word processors and electric typewriters should be investigated before a purchase is made.

8

Microcomputers for word processing and graphics

People must understand that science is
inherently neither a potential for good nor
for evil. It is a potential to be harnessed
by man to do his bidding.

Glenn T. Seaborg (1964)

In recent years microcomputers have become available which are suitable for industrial, educational and domestic use. Over the years their cost has reduced so that their purchase has become a realistic proposition for use in a wide range of situations. Cost, however, remains such that careful thought and consideration is needed before deciding to invest in the necessary pieces of equipment, particularly if the purchase is for a sole user.

It would not be wise to recommend particular systems for purchase because individual needs vary so much. The facilities which are ideal for one user may not suit another. Similarly, the physical characteristics of some pieces of equipment will suit some users more than others. A further reason for not suggesting particular systems is that microcomputing facilities develop at a rapid rate; a system that is new to the market this year will be replaced by a later model during the following year, if not during the following months.

This rapid development of new systems and facilities can make purchase difficult. Systems are considered, decisions almost made, then news breaks that in x months a revolutionary system will be available. This will happen no matter when the decision is made, there will always be some 'better' system being developed for the market. Unless that system will have facilities which will be of great advantage to the user, one should make an informed choice from what is currently available; procrastination could continue indefinitely.

CONSIDERATIONS WHEN CHOOSING THE EQUIPMENT

For the reasons described above it is not advisable to recommend specific pieces of equipment, but some general considerations will help in the choice of system.

1. Will the system be used only for word processing or are other microcomputer facilities required? If the system is to be used solely for word processing, a package incorporating a micro-computer, disk drives, visual display unit (VDU) and printer may be purchased at a relatively small cost. Should the equipment be required for other purposes, for example graphic work, a micro-computer in which a word processing chip is inserted plus, of course, the other necessary pieces of equipment will probably form a more suitable purchase.
2. Will the equipment be used only by one person or will it, for instance, be used by a number of members of the family? Each user may employ it for a different function, so that a more versatile machine may be required than if it was to be used only by one person.
3. Are there friends or colleagues who also use microcomputers? It is useful to have a system which is compatible with that of other users so that programs and disks may be loaned or exchanged. Should the user be a child or a student attending an educational establishment, it would be best to select equipment which is compatible with that being used in school or college. For example, at present, most British schools use BBC microcomputers. A microcomputer used in the home or for therapy in a clinical setting by a student will be most useful if it is compatible with the one used in school, so that similar programs may be used in all situations and the user has only to become accustomed to using one type of equipment.
4. Before any decision is reached about purchasing equipment careful consideration should be given to the functions and types of programs which will be required. The first consideration should be the software required. Look at the programs which will be needed and ones which are likely to be needed in the future, then select the microcomputer which will run them. Many people make the mistake of buying a microcomputer then finding that the types of program they wish to use are not available for their chosen machine. Always decide on the types of programs which will be required together with the required computing facilities,

127

then choose the system which fulfils these needs. If a micro-computer is already being used in an educational establishment or therapeutically in a medical establishment take advice from the experts in these places. Alternatively, visit centres which have been set up to provide information about microcomputing equipment for educational, communication or therapeutic purposes. Should advice be sought from a retail outlet ensure that a large range of equipment is stocked or can be easily obtained. An outlet which sells only a limited range of equipment is more likely to advise purchase from that range, which may not be the most suitable for the intended use. Always ensure that the user has ample 'hands on' experience before deciding to make a purchase.

THE EQUIPMENT

A number of pieces of equipment are necessary for microcomputing. Many other pieces of sophisticated equipment may be added to the basic list which increase the facilities of the microcomputer. The following list includes the minimum of equipment which will be required.

1. Hardware
   (a) The microcomputer and the keyboard are usually combined in one unit. Sometimes the keyboard is a separate unit which may be an advantage for those users who wish to support the keyboard on their lap or on the small tray attached to a wheelchair.
   (b) The monitor or VDU provides a visual display output from the microcomputer.
   (c) The disk drive or cassette recorder records information on disk or tape.
   (d) The printer.
2. Software
   (a) Disks or tapes on which information is stored and from which it may be retrieved.
   (b) Paper for the printer.

Microcomputer

Check the position of the on/off switch. Is it in a position which is accessible to the user? Is it of a type which the user can activate?

Check the position of user ports. These are sockets into which additional pieces of equipment may be plugged, such as special switching devices for users unable to use the keyboard. Are they in an easily accessible position? This is particularly important if the sockets are used for a number of different devices and need to be connected and disconnected frequently.

Keyboard

Most keyboards are arranged in the traditional QWERTY layout, similar to that of a typewriter, with additional keys which are used for computing and word processing.

Some of the cheaper keyboards are very small, much smaller than a conventional typewriter. Unless there are special reasons for needing a small keyboard, for instance because movement is very limited, they are not very comfortable to use, especially for people who are accustomed to conventional keyboards.

The keys on some keyboards are made of soft plastic which provides little resistance and gives no indication of when the key has fired, which makes touch typing difficult and could require frequent reference to the VDU to ascertain that the required function has taken place.

On many of the smaller keyboards each key has as many as four functions, lower case letters, upper case letters which also require the depression of the shift key and two other functions which require the additional depression of special function keys. This entails learning additional manoeuvres in order to use the keyboard effectively, as well as requiring a greater number of two handed movements which may be difficult or even impossible for some people.

Some keyboards have flat keys which are adequate for computing but are not comfortable for extended pieces of word processing. If word processing is the main function for which the keyboard will be used the keys should be dished, i.e. be slightly concave so that the fingers fit comfortable on them.

Monitor (VDU)

Some dedicated word processor have 7 inch screens (measured diagonally) others have 12 inch screens. Some users may find that an even larger screen is better suited to their needs. It should be noted that the size of the screen does not usually influence the amount of information or text which may be displayed; this is usually controlled by the program which is being used.

The material may be displayed in white, green or amber against a black background or a colour monitor may be used. Look at the various combinations of colours on a variety of screens before purchasing, for some colours may appear clearer and easier on the eye of the user.

Investigate also the clarity of the display. This will depend on the resolution – the number of lines of the screen. A VDU manufactured as a monitor for a microcomputer will have a higher resolution and is therefore infinitely more suitable for word processing or any other microcomputing than a screen used for viewing television. It is false economy to employ the family television set as a VDU, for it will not be comfortable to scan at close range for prolonged periods. Nor will the microcomputer be popular with the other members of the family if their television viewing is thus restricted.

The VDU will have contrast and brightness controls which may be adjusted to suit the user. Whenever possible these and the on/off control should be within easy reach of the user. The type of control, e.g. a knob to twist, button to push, lever to move left to right or top to bottom, should be chosen to suit the hand function of the user. It may be possible to enlarge or alter the shape of control buttons or switches with two part epoxy resins modelled into a suitable shape on the button or switch.

Anti-glare screens may be fitted over the VDU screen, these are reported to reduce visual discomfort resulting from prolonged use. Screen filters are also available which are reported to polarize incoming light and trap reflected light, suppressing the glare from windows and lights and thus enhancing the contrast of the screen.

It may be that ocular discomfort is experienced when using a VDU for prolonged periods. This may occur because the user concentrates on the screen and does not blink as frequently as usual and so the eyeball is not lubricated. A conscious effort to blink frequently will probably solve or reduce the discomfort.

Storage devices

Material may be stored on and retrieved from a cassette of magnetic tape or a disk.

Tape

It is possible to record material on a magnetic tape by means of a cassette recorder. It is a cheaper method than using a disk and disk drive but not nearly so convenient. Tapes are slow to use. There is no random access; the tape must be run until the required material is found. They are easily corrupted, resulting in loss of stored material. A very limited amount of material may be stored on one tape so that far more handling of tape cassettes is required than when data is stored on disks.

The amount of handling of equipment which is required is an important consideration for those with limited hand and arm function. The advantages of using cassette tapes to store material are few, other than cheapness. Magnetic tape is, however, enclosed in a rigid cassette and is thus easier to handle than a floppy disk. Even this advantage is being superseded by the newer floppy disks which are enclosed in a rigid case.

Disks

Material may also be recorded on disks by means of a disk drive which may be an integral part of a word processor or a separate unit. Disk drives may be single, housing one disk at a time, or double, capable of housing two disks. A double disk drive is useful when copying material from one disk to another. It is possible to do this with a single disk drive but it is a longer process and involves more loading and unloading of disks which may be a difficult procedure for some people.

Most systems use either a 5.25 inch or 3.5 inch disk, both of which are housed in a protective cover. The smaller size of disk is capable of holding more text than the larger one. For a person who finds it difficult to remove and insert disks independently the consideration of the amount of material which may be stored on a disk is an important one.

A further advantage of the smaller size of disk is that it is enclosed in a rigid protective cover which provides better protection from accidental damage and also makes it easier to insert and remove from the disk drive.

A third type of disk is the hard disk which is never removed from its drive. This type of disk will hold many thousands of pages of text, as much as many people will ever need to store. For the person with impaired hand function the advantages are manifold. The disadvantage is the high cost of such disks.

Whichever type of storage device is used, it is important that material is well organized and catalogued. Initially this may seem unnecessary but eventually a large amount of material will be stored and, unless it is well catalogued, the retrieval of information will become an irksome task.

Printers

The type of printer chosen will depend on the personal taste of the user and the type of material which will be printed. Two types of printer are most frequently used – dot matrix and daisy wheel.

Dot matrix printers

The printing head consists of a series of pins, a number of which are selected to print particular characters by striking the ribbon which is situated between the printer head and the paper.

Advantages of dot matrix printers

1. Many models are less expensive than daisy wheel printers.
2. They print very quickly, usually between 80 and 200 characters per second (cps). Unless the printer is being used commercially, this speed is rarely a necessity.
3. They may be used to print graphics as well as different sizes and styles of print. This facility is useful for printing news sheets, posters and the like. Large print may be important if the printer is used by young children or people with visual impairment.
4. Some models allow print styles to be changed within a document, e.g. from roman to italic.

Disadvantages of dot matrix printers

1. Because the print is formed by a series of dots it is not solid. The printed text will therefore not be as clear as that produced by a

daisy wheel printer. This quality will be significant for people with impaired vision. There are of course various qualities of dot matrix printer, some having more pins on the print head than others. The more pins entailed in forming a character the more solid the print will appear. Examining a sample of text through a magnifying glass allows the solidity of the print to be assessed more clearly. With many printers the definition of the print may be enhanced by using the double strike facility. As the term suggests this causes each letter character to be printed twice, the second time exactly on top of the first. This process does, of course mean that each page takes longer to print.

2. The pins on the printing head of many dot matrix printers are arranged in a rectangle, e.g. 5 by 7 or 7 by 9 pins. With this arrangement it is difficult to produce true descenders for lower case letter characters such as g, y and p. This may reduce the clarity of these characters. It may also be significant for children who use a word processor for some of their written work because of difficulties with handwriting. Such children frequently have problems with the relative size of letter characters and spatial relationship to each other. The lack of true descenders could re-inforce these difficulties.

Top quality dot matrix printers often produce print of very nearly the standard of a daisy wheel printer.

Daisy wheel printers

This type of printer is intended only for printing letter and number characters; it cannot be used to reproduce graphics. The characters are arranged on the spokes of a wheel (hence the name daisy wheel) which spins until the required character is in the correct position to be printed.

Advantages of daisy wheel printers

1. The print is solid and therefore very clear and easy to read.
2. Lower case letter characters have true descenders which means that letter characters are printed in the correct proportions and positions to each other.

Disadvantages of daisy wheel printers

1. These printers are usually more expensive than the dot matrix type.

2. They print relatively slowly, usually between 12 and 55 cps. In practice this would only be a problem for people who intend using their word processing skills for business purposes where speed is important. For most other people these speeds are adequate.
3. Unless the printing is halted and the daisy wheel changed, it is not possible to change the style of print within a document.
4. It is not possible to print graphics with a daisy wheel printer.

Printer ribbons

Ribbons for most printers are enclosed in a cassette which makes them simple to insert. Insertion does not require precise finger/ thumb apposition. The ribbon is not exposed, so that removing and inserting them does not soil the hands. There are a number of types of ribbon. Before purchasing a printer check the types of ribbon which are available for it. Some types are more expensive to use than others.

1. *Carbon ribbon – single strike* They produce good quality, clearly defined print. The ribbon moves so that each character is printed on a fresh section of the ribbon. This is the most expensive type of ribbon to use because it passes only once before the print head.

2. *Carbon ribbon – multi-strike* This type of ribbon has the qualities of the single strike ribbon except that the ribbon moves only fractionally for each successive character which is printed. It is therefore more economical to use.

3. *Fabric ribbon* These ribbons may be used many times, the resultant print will become less dense with each re-use of the ribbon. Even the first run of the ribbon will not produce as clearly defined print as that produced by carbon ribbon, however fabric ribbons are economical to use for first drafts and other work where the appearance of the printed page is not of paramount importance. Because the ribbons may be used many times without attention they are useful for people who have a large print output but lack the manual dexterity to remove and insert ribbons.

Paper

Paper in one of three forms may be used: single sheet, fan fold or roll.

1. Single sheets of paper may be fed by hand into the printer. The user therefore has a wide choice of the types of paper used, including headed notepaper or perhaps different colours of paper within the same piece of work. For those unable to insert single sheets it is possible to buy a cut-sheet feeder which will automatically feed single sheets of paper into the printer. Single sheet feeders are available as an optional extra for most daisy wheel printers. They tend to be expensive.
2. Fan fold paper is usually fed into the printer by means of a tractor feed. The paper has a row of holes close to each edge which fit on to the tractor mechanism. The paper is also perforated so that it may be torn into separate sheets if required. This method of feeding paper into the printer will be helpful for people who are unable to feed paper into the printer independently but the long continuous sheet limits the choice of type of paper which may be used. The holes down the edge of the paper are often located on a perforated strip which may be removed from the paper after printing. The smoothness of the edges of the paper will depend on the size of the perforations.
3. Rolls of paper may be used with a friction feed printer which will also take single sheets of paper. The roll of unused paper needs some device to control it.

WORD PROCESSING PACKAGES

Chapter 6 contains a section on the use of microcomputers in artwork, graphics and technical drawing. The remainder of this chapter, therefore, concentrates on the use of microcomputers for recording words on paper.

Packages are available which contain the equipment necessary for word processing; dedicated word processors. They are not usually suitable to be used for other microcomputing purposes. They are however relatively cheap and a good purchase for those who are absolutely sure that other facilities will not be required at present or in the foreseeable future.

Another way to obtain word processing facilities is by means of microcomputing equipment to which a word processing element is added. This addition may be a word processing program contained on a disk. It is possible to use such a program with only a single disk drive. The disk must be inserted into the drive and loaded into the computer then the disk must be replaced with the working disk, the disk on which text will be stored. For people with severe impairment of hand function for whom inserting and removing disks from the drive is difficult, a double disk drive is preferable, whereby the disk containing the word processing program is housed in one drive and the working disk in the other thus removing the need for frequent handling of disks.

A second method of obtaining word processing facilities is by means of a word processing chip which is fitted in one of the ports inside the computer. This is a good method of providing word processing facilities because the facility is always ready for use without having to manipulate any pieces of equipment; it will only be necessary to access the facility by typing in the appropriate code. There is not a great deal of difference between the cost of these two systems.

A wide variety of word processing programs are available, the choice being limited, of course, by their compatibility with the microcomputer which is to be used. Compatibility of program and microcomputer is essential.

Programs vary from simple ones with which very young children may record a few words to very complex ones intended for use by people who produce large amounts of text for their own and commercial uses. One very simple program provides strips on which the letter characters are displayed. Both the colour of the strips and the colour of the letter characters may be selected to provide the most easily seen colour contrast for the user. This program is only intended for very small amounts of work.

Other simple programs available are suitable for recording several pages of work in which large characters are displayed on the VDU as well as when printed on paper. These are uncomplicated programs which have the minimum of editing commands. There is a large selection of word processing programs available, the choice being governed by the type of microcomputer which will run them and the personal taste of the user. Some programs can be mastered within a few days, others, usually those with many facilities, take longer to learn to use proficiently. While it is pointless acquiring a program containing facilities which will never be used, before purchase consideration should be given to the facilities which may be required in the future. There is no substitute for hands on experience and it is strongly advised that the user of the program has it thoroughly demonstrated and actually tries using it before purchase.

How then is a microcomputer with a word processing facility superior to a typewriter, especially for people with a motor disability?

Advantages of word processors

1. Words will be recorded more quickly because mistakes are instantly rectifiable. There is no need to be nervous about compiling a perfect copy of a piece of work. Spelling and grammar are correctable before the copy is printed.
2. It is possible to think whilst using a word processing program. A piece of work may originate as only a few key words and be expanded as desired. Because the work is recorded on a disk it is possible to record the piece of work in a semi-finished state and return to it at any time in the future. It is not a disaster if after a piece of work has been printed a mistake is discovered. The necessary correction is made to the document, the revised text recorded on disk to replace the inaccurate one and the corrected text printed without the need to use correction fluid or retype the entire piece as would be necessary if using a typewriter.
3. Layouts may be prepared for standard letters, stored on disk and used as required for individual letters when only the body of the letter will need to be added. This facility is particularly useful for people who because of motor dysfunction find recording even using a word processor a long process.

Disadvantages of word processors

1. Word processing packages may be bought for the price of an expensive office model typewriter. They cost more than many people would intend paying for a typewriter.
2. Except for the very expensive portable machines primarily intended for business people to use whilst travelling, the equipment needed to run a word processing program is not portable. It is usually best to have the equipment set up in a position where it is immediately ready for use. Should the equipment need to be

set up on every occasion it is used, in many instances it will only be used infrequently.

LEARNING TO USE A WORD PROCESSOR

In a similar way to any other keyboard, the user must learn keyboard layout and appropriate fingering. The fingering adopted will, of course, vary according to the abilities of the user. A young child may use a picture method, an older one a simplified version of a typing program, others will need to adapt fingering according to the number of digits which may be used (see Chapter 7).

In addition to these conventional methods of learning the keyboard many word processing programs have supplied with them a program for teaching keyboard skills. Some people are happy to use such a program alone in order to become proficient. Others will find that this solitary process lacks in motivation. Perhaps the best system is to use such a program in conjunction with personal tuition to provide motivation, prevent the development of bad fingering habits and to deal with any functional and perceptual difficulties.

ADDITIONAL FACILITIES PROVIDED BY A WORD PROCESSING PROGRAM

Storage and retrieval

Pieces of work may be stored on disk or tape at any point and retrieved when required so that they may be completed or amended.

Review of text

Long texts may be reviewed on the monitor, rather than read from paper, which removes the need to separate and turn individual sheets of paper.

Menu facilities

Word processing programs are provided with a 'menu' which provides for the instant use of a number of facilities. These facilities will vary according to the program being used. The menu facilities available may include, saving text on to a disk or tape and ready retrieval of that text. It may also be possible to save on disk or tape only part of the text in the microcomputer memory by marking the required piece of text. Two pieces of text may be merged into one document.

By using the 'search and replace' item from the menu, it is possible to change a particular word throughout a text. For example, it may be decided that the name, Mark, is not suitable for the hero of a story and that David is more apt. This facility allows all the occurrences of 'Mark' to be instantly replaced by 'David'.

Care must be taken, for should 'Mark' be used in another context, for example, 'Mark my word', that occurrence of 'Mark' will also be replaced by 'David', the phrase then reading 'David my word'.

Some word processing programs display on the VDU the text exactly as it will be printed (WYSIWYG – what you see is what you get). Other systems which do not have this facility provide a menu item which allows the user to see the layout of the text as it will be printed. Printing the text is often a menu facility which, provided the printer is switched on and paper inserted, requires only the firing of one or perhaps two keys.

Cursor

The cursor, the flashing marker on the VDU, is used in word processing to denote the point in the text at which the next character key to be fired will be shown on the screen. The cursor is controlled by keys which allow it to be moved to left or right, up or down. This facility allows text to be inserted wherever it is required. For instance, if it is found that necessary has been spelt 'necesary', moving the cursor to the point where a second s is to be added will allow the spelling to be corrected. Using this method it is not only possible to insert single letter characters but also phrases, sentences, paragraphs or even longer pieces of text.

By using the cursor key in the appropriate position it is also possible, by also using the delete key to remove letters, words or longer sections of text.

Function keys

Most word processing programs employ the function keys of the microcomputer to provide instant additional facilities. These facilities will vary between programs. Some of the following facilities may be provided.

1. The choice between inserting extra text and overwriting text which has already been written.
2. The insertion of markers at two specific points in the text so that the text between the markers may be deleted, moved *en bloc* to the position denoted by the cursor or copied at the cursor position by firing another function key.
3. Another function key will provide a word count of a portion of text the beginning of which is denoted by the cursor and the end by a character not used in the text.

Layout and editing

A word processor will also be of great help in arranging the layout of completed text. Many of the details of layout which have to be prepared manually when using a conventional typewriter can be set at the beginning of or, as needed, within text without the need to make judgements regarding spacing and the like. Moreover should the layout later prove to be unsatisfactory there is no need to retype the complete text; the desired alterations may be made to the commands which control layout and the original text reprinted in its new format.

The editing commands which are available will, of course, vary between the various programs which are available. The following is a list of the most commonly available commands.

1. The left margin may be set at the required width.
2. Unlike a printed page in a book, the right hand margin of a page of typed material will be ragged, words at the end of each line will not finish the same number of spaces from the edge of the paper. Many word processing programs allow the right hand margin to be straight like a page of print in a book. This is achieved by adjusting the spaces between words in each line of text so that the last letters of each line are exactly underneath each other. This facility is especially useful when preparing

information sheets, leaflets and the like (Figure 7.2).

3. When preparing text with a conventional typewriter there is usually an auditory signal to indicate when the end of a line is near and the typist must judge whether or not to begin typing a new word on that line or whether a word may be successfully divided between that line and the next. Word processing removes the need for this personal judgement. By setting the desired length of lines at the beginning of a piece of work, the user need not be concerned with line length for the program will arrange line ends automatically.

4. The program will also take care of the number of lines which will be printed on each page as well as the amount of space at the top and bottom of each page.

5. The number of spaces between each line of text may be set by the appropriate command at the beginning of a piece of work. This spacing may be altered if desired at any point within a text. Wide spaces between lines will be useful both on the VDU and on the printed page for people who have difficulty scanning lines of print on a closely printed page such as those who have difficulty with figure/background discrimination. Wide spaces between lines of print are also helpful for children who are only used to reading pages with a few lines of widely spaced text.

6. Centring a title or other material on the page requires precise calculation on the part of the user when using a conventional typewriter. A word processing program only requires the centring command to be inserted in the appropriate position in the text, no calculation on the part of the user is necessary.

7. Pages of text may be numbered in sequence if desired.

8. Tabulation is much easier than with a conventional typewriter. The appropriate command at the beginning of a piece of text makes the firing of the tabulation key the only manoeuvre necessary to produce columns of text (Figure 8.1).

9. Facilities may be incorporated into some word processing programs, presented on a separate disk or contained on a chip which is fitted to one of the ports inside the microcomputer, which will check the spelling of a text which is loaded in the microcomputer. Ensure that the spelling checker program is compatible with the word processing program which is being used should the two be purchased as separate items.

The size of the vocabulary contained in these programs varies. It is possible to add a personally useful vocabulary to some programs. When in use the program will proof read a document,

Figure 8.1: An example of embedded commands used to produce tabulated text.

```
f1  LL50  f1  LM10  f1  DT10,15,30  f2
```

1.	Line length	50
2.	Left margin	10
3.	First tab.	10
4.	Second tab.	15
5.	Third tab.	30

mark what, according to the program's dictionary, are errors and suggest alternative possibilities of correct spellings. It should be noted that a spelling checker will only mark incorrect spelling, it will not differentiate between homophones. 'Steal' and 'steel', 'there' and 'their' are spelled correctly, a spelling checker will not inform the user which of each pair of spellings is correct in a particular instance for it does not correct grammar or the meaning of sentences.

It cannot be stressed too strongly that no amount of reading or demonstrations of word processing programs can compensate for actual hands on experience. Many processes which appear complex when read from the page are simple when put into practice. Demonstrations of programs can seem baffling when many facilities are demonstrated during a single session. Before decisions are made about the purchase of a system ensure that the proposed user has sufficient personal experience working with the program to be sure that a suitable one is being purchased.

SPECIAL ADVANTAGES OF WORD PROCESSING FOR CHILDREN WHO HAVE HANDWRITING DIFFICULTIES

Children are much less wary of microcomputers than adults. Even very young children will quickly learn how to operate simple programs and will accept computer logic with ease. Those who have used games and educational programs will usually adapt to using word processing programs (Hope, 1980).

Should it be decided that word processing is a beneficial method for a child to record on paper a systematic method of teaching keyboard skills should be initiated (Chapter 7). On no account should the child be allowed to search for and strike keys in a haphazard manner.

Many of the advantages of word processing for children are similar to those experienced by adults, as described earlier. Young children, being in the process of attaining lexical skills, obtain other advantages which occur from the use of word processing.

1. Most children are familiar with microcomputers, they are less nervous of attempting word processing than of using a conventional typewriter with which they are not so familiar.
2. Because the text displayed on the VDU is instantly correctable, children are more enthusiastic about attempting to spell words they are not completely familiar with, as well as composing sentences and ordering pieces of work.
3. The correction work is not so traumatic for the child because it may be done whilst the text is displayed on the screen and before it is printed. The piece of work is not spoiled by corrections and ultimately the child possesses a perfect piece of work.
4. It is an ideal medium for group work because the work may begin from a brief outline which is subsequently expanded, or alternatively from ideas displayed on the VDU generated from a brainstorming session. The whole group may monitor on the VDU what each member is currently typing. Peer help can be given with spellings and sentence construction. The piece of work may be expanded or rearranged to the satisfaction of all group members. Ultimately a united printed piece of work will be produced.

SPECIAL DEVICES TO ENABLE PEOPLE WITH IMPAIRED HAND FUNCTION TO USE A MICROCOMPUTER

The previous chapter describes some of the devices which may be used to fire the keys of the keyboard, such as typing sticks and head sticks. It also contains details of other measures which may be taken to help the keyboard user who has disabilities to work more comfortably and efficiently. There are also suggestions regarding the use of scanning devices, expanded and mini-keyboards. These devices and adaptations can, of course, also be used by people using a micro-computer keyboard.

A microcomputer can, by the addition of special switching devices, become accessible to those with severe motor disability. A variety of switching devices is commercially available and, where necessary, devices may be designed to suit the specific needs of an individual user. It is possible to design controls which are activated by almost any part of the body.

1. Touch switches of various designs are available. They consist of a switch plate which as its name suggests, is activated by touch. Their size can be adjusted to suit the user, the area of contact being large for those with inaccurate movement. The sensitivity of the switch can be adjusted to respond to the lightest touch.
2. Pressure pads are operated by pressing the soft top. They may be flat for those who can only raise the hand a very small distance above the height of the table on which it is resting. Other pressure pads are deeper and do not provide such a large area of contact.
3. There are a number of types of stick device. Wobble sticks for those with very little controlled movements are activated by knocking in any direction. Joysticks have a minimum of two functions activated by either pushing and pulling forwards and backwards or to the left and right. Others have up to eight functions activated by the direction in which the joystick is moved.
4. Foot switches are designed for both people who are able to precisely control movement and those who have only gross movement.
5. Pressure switches may be suitably mounted so that they may be activated by almost any part of the body. For example by moving the head from side to side or lowering the chin onto the switch.
6. Very sensitive touch switches which may be mounted on spectacle frames or a headband are activated by the tongue. Other mouth switches are operated by a suck and puff input.
7. Reflected beam switches may be activated by eye movement or by blinking for a specified length of time.

Many types of switching devices are commercially available or can be manufactured to fill specific needs. Expert advice is necessary when selecting the most appropriate device (Heddell, 1985; Nelham, 1988; Saunders, 1984). Ideally the client should visit a centre which specializes in such equipment and where the staff have wide experience of such equipment and the needs and problems of users. The staff will be able to suggest systems which are most likely to be appropriate. Such centres have displays of at least a selection of the equipment available, which may be tested by the client before a purchase is made.

OTHER MICRO PROCESSING EQUIPMENT WHICH MAY BE USED TO RECORD ON PAPER

Portable word processors

There are several types of small portable word processors which are battery powered such as the Microscribe and the Sharp Memowriter (Figure 8.2). These machines are light enough to hold on the lap or the tray of a wheelchair. Because of their small size these machines have small keys and are not suitable for use by people who have poorly coordinated hand movements.

The Memowriter has a display which shows up to 20 letters so that corrections may be made before text is printed. Text, up to 20 letters per line, is printed on paper contained on a roll.

The Microscribe has a memory of 8000 characters. Text may be sent to a printer by means of an interface.

Microwriter

The Microwriter, a portable word processor, was originally designed to be used by business people but has been found to be suitable for use by some people with limited hand function (Figure 8.3). It is operated by using various combinations of its five keys. Because there is only a single key for each digit, the hand, once in position, is not moved. Machines are available with key arrangements for both left and right-handed users.

The Microwriter may be adapted to satisfy special needs, such as a stiff keyboard for people with a mild tremor, re-arranged keys to suit individual needs and a sequential version to use with a head pointer or other device. The Quinkey, a keyboard-only version of the Microwriter, can be used to activate the keys of a micro-computer. Up to four Quinkeys may input into one microcomputer, making it a useful device for group work in a classroom.

Figure 8.2: An example of a small, lightweight word processor.

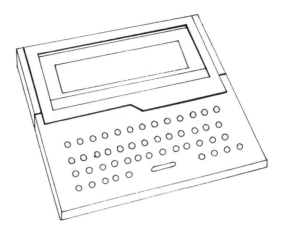

Figure 8.3: The Microwriter.

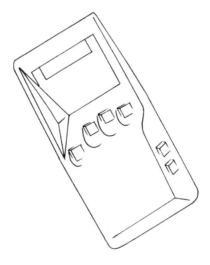

CONCLUSION

The development of microcomputers continues apace. Facilities are constantly being refined and are becoming increasingly user friendly. The cost of equipment has been reduced considerably in recent years. A generation of children is growing up in a world of micro-computing.

Therapists, teachers, electronic engineers and computer programmers are becoming increasingly interested in the needs of people with disabilities and the benefit they can gain from microcomputing facilities. Perhaps it is not too idealistic to envisage the day when everyone who could benefit from the use of a microcomputer will have ready access to one.

References

Alston, J. and Taylor, J. (1987) *Handwriting: Theory, Research and Practice*, Croom Helm, London, p. 12.

Ayres, A.J. (1974) *The Development of Sensory Integration Theory and Practice*, Kendall/Hunt Publishing Company, Dubuque, Iowa, p. 4.

Barzun (1976) *The International Theraurus of Quotations* (ed. R. Thomas Tripp), Penguin, London, p. 33.

Beecher, H.W. (1976) *The International Theraurus of Quotations* (ed. R. Thomas Tripp), Penguin, London, p. 712.

Blakemore, C. (1988) *The Mind Machine*, BBC Publications, London, pp. 2–3.

Bobath, K. (1974) *The Motor Deficit of Patients with Cerebral Palsy*, Spastics International Medical Publications/Heinemann Medical Books, London, pp. 7–10.

Bowley, A.H. (1969) in *Cerebral Palsy and the Young Child* (ed. S. Blencoe), E. & S. Livingstone, Edinburgh, p. 103.

Burr, L.A. (1980) Use of vision in the function of hand eye co-ordination. *British Journal of Occupational Therapy*, **43** (2) 59–63.

Chapman, L.J., Lewis, A. and Wedell, K. (1970) A note on reversals in the writing of eight-year-old children. *Remedial Education*, **5** (2) 91–4.

Chasty, H.T. (1986) Handwriting a suitable approach for the child with difficulty. Lecture/Handwriting Interest Group, September.

Craft, A.W. (1985) Arthritis in children. *British Journal of Hospital Medicine*, **33** (4) 188–94.

Crooks, M. (undated) *Special Typewriter Keyboard Charts and Instructions for Handicapped Typists*, Committee for Writing and Reading Aids for the Paralysed, National Fund for Research into Crippling Diseases, Vincent House, Springfield Road, Horsham, Sussex RH12 2PN.

Deacon, J.J. (1974) *Tongue Tied. Fifty years of friendship in a subnormality hospital*, National Society for Mentally Handicapped Children, Pembroke Hall, Pembroke Square, London.

Enstrom, E.A. (1974) The extent of the use of the left hand in handwriting. *Journal of Educational Research*, **55** (5) 234–5.

Fahn, S. (1972) Differential diagnosis of tremors. *Symposium on Clinical Neurology*, **56** (6) 1363–75.

Frankenburg, W.K. and Dodds, J.B. (1969) *Denver Developmental Screening Test*, University of Colorado Medical Center, Denver.

Fraser, K. (1985) *Word Processing and Typing*, Usborne Publishing, London.

Goad, M. (1977) A picture approach to typewriting. *Special Education – Forward Trends*, **4** (1) 14–16.

Guiard, Y. and Millerat, F. (1984) Writing postures of left-handers: inverters are hand-crossers. *Neuropsychologia*, **22** (4) 535–8.

Heddell, T. (1985) *With a Little Help from the Chip*, BBC Publications, London.

Herodotus (1976) *The International Theraurus of Quotations* (ed. R. Thomas Tripp), Penguin, London, 1976, p. 582.

Herxheimer, A. (ed.) (1988) Dystonia: undiagnosed and undertreated? *Drug and Therapeutics Bulletin*, **26** (9) 33–6.

Hope, M. (1980) How can microcomputers help? *Special Education – Forward Trends*, **7** (4) 14–16.

Illingworth, R.S. (1983) *The Development of the Infant and Young Child: Normal and Abnormal*, 7th Edition, Churchill Livingstone, Edinburgh, p. 159.

Illingworth, R.S. and Illingworth, C. (1984) *Babies and Young Children; A Guide for Parents*, Churchill Livingstone, Edinburgh, p. 118.

Janitch, V. (1975) *Country Collage*, Ward Lock, London.

Jarman, C. (1984) Pre-handwriting activities for young children. *Gnosis*, **5**, 26–8.

Johnson, W., Schwartz, G. and Barbeau, A. (1962) Studies on dystonia musculorum deformans. *Archives of Neurology*, **7**, 301–13.

Kipling, R. Just So Stories, *The Practical Encyclopedia for Children*, Odhams Press Ltd, London, reprinted 1947 (original date of publication not stated) frontispiece.

Levy, J. and Reid, M. (1976) Variations in writing posture and cerebral organisation. *Science*, **194**, 337–8.

Mulcahy, C. (1986) An approach to the assessment of sitting ability for the prescription of seating. *British Journal of Occupational Therapy*, **49** (11) 367–8.

Mulcahy, C.M., Poultney, T.E., Nelham, R.L., Green, E.M. and Billington, G.D. (1988) Adaptive seating for motor handicap: problems, a solution, assessment and prescription. *British Journal of Occupational Therapy*, **51** (10) 347–52.

Myers, Prue Wallis (1987) The sloping board. *Handwriting Review*, **1**, 43.

Nelham, R.L. (1988) *Assistive Devices*, Rehabilitation Engineering Unit, Chailey Heritage, North Chailey, nr Lewes, East Sussex, BN8 4EF.

Nolan, C. (1981) *Dam-burst of Dreams*, Pan Books, London.

Nolan, C. (1987) *Under the Eye of the Clock*, Weidenfeld and Nicholson, London.

O'Hare, A.E. and Brown, J.K. (1989) Childhood dysgraphia. Part 1, An illustrated clinical classification. *Child: Care, Health and Development*, **15** (2) 79–104.

Osborne, T. (1987) Flexy Computer Trolley. *British Journal of Occupational Therapy*, **50** (11) 11.

Parry, M. (1977) *Stenciling*, Litton Educational Publishing, New York.

Penso, D.E. (1987) *Occupational Therapy for Children with Disabilities*, Croom Helm, London, pp. 131–71.

Pluckrose, H. (1967) *Introducing Crayon Techniques*, Batsford, London.

Richardson, N.K. (1959) *Type With One Hand*, South Western Publishing, USA.

Rockey, J. and Nelham, R.L. (1984) Seating for the chairbound child in *The Physically Handicapped Child* (ed. G.T. McCarthy), Faber and Faber, London.

Saunders, P. (1984) *Micros for Handicapped Users*, Helena Press, Orchard Land, Goathland, Whitby, North Yorks. YO22 5JT.

Scott, G. (1973) *Introducing Finger Painting*, Batsford, London.

Seaborg, G.T. (1976) *The International Theraurus of Quotations* (ed.

R. Thomas Tripp), Penguin, London, p. 563.

Sheridan, M.D. (1975) *From Birth to Five Years*, NFER-Nelson.

Thomas, D. (1967) The hand that signed the paper, in *Poetry of the 1930s* (ed. A. Rodway), Longman, Green and Co. Ltd, London and Harlow, p. 152.

Vernon, M.D. (1971) *The Psychology of Perception*, Penguin, London.

Workman, D., Geggie, C. and Creasey, G. (1988) The microcomputer as an aid to written communication. *British Journal of Occupational Therapy*, **51** (6) 188–90.

Ziviani, J. (1982) Children's prehension while writing, a pilot study. *British Journal of Occupational Therapy*, **45** (5) 306–7.

Further reading

Allin, R.E. and Lawson, D.S. (1977) *The Management of Juvenile Chronic Polyarthritis*, The Association of Paediatric Chartered Physiotherapists, P.C.P. Publications, Crawley, West Sussex.

Alston, J. (1985) Brittle bones: a handicap with special occupational therapy needs. *British Journal of Occupational Therapy*, **48** (4) 103–5.

Alston, J. and Taylor, J. (1985) *Helping Left Handed Children with Handwriting: Interpreting Research for Teachers and Therapists* (Supplement to the Handwriting File), LDA, Wisbech, Cambs.

Alston, J. and Taylor, J. (1988) *Handwriting File*, 2nd edn, LDA, Wisbech, Cambs.

Anderson, E.M. (1976) Impairment of motor (manual skill) in children with spina bifida myelomeningocele and hydrocephalus. *British Journal of Occupational Therapy*, **39** (4) 91–3.

Anderson, E.M. and Cambridge, J. (1979) Helping spina bifida hydrocephalus pupils with handwriting. *Special Education – Forward Trends*, **6** (1) 15–17.

Armstrong, J. and Rennie, J. (1986) We can use computers too! The setting up of a project for mentally handicapped residents. *British Journal of Occupational Therapy*, **49** (9) 297–300.

Belkin, G.S. (1984) *How to Start and Run Your Own Word-Processing Business*, John Wiley & Sons, New York.

Benjamin, W. (1987) Craft design technology. Suitable software for creative classrooms. *A & B Computing*, **4** (9) 96–100.

Bishop, D.V.M. (1980) Handedness, Clumsiness and Cognitive Ability. *Developmental Medicine and Child Neurology*, **22**, 569–79.

Bishop, D.V.M. (1984) Using non-preferred hand skill to investigate pathological left-handedness in an unselected population. *Developmental Medicine and Child Neurology*, **26**, 214–26.

Boleach, J. (1986) *Stencilling with Style*, David and Charles, Newton Abbot.

Chambers, H.T. (1982) *Making the Most of Word Processing*, Business Books, Hutchinson, London.

Clark, M.M. (1974) *Teaching Left-handed Children*, Hodder & Stoughton, Sevenoaks, Kent.

Consumer Association Ltd (1987) Homebanking. *Which?* October, pp. 463.

Consumer Association Ltd (1987) Home in on a computer. *Which?* November, pp. 526–9.

Consumer Association Ltd (1987) Picking a word processing package. *Which?* December, pp. 600–1.

Consumer Association Ltd (1988) Computers for home use. *Which?* November, pp. 523–7.

Craft, A.W. (1985) Arthritis in children. *British Journal of Hospital Medicine*, **33** (4) 188–94.

Curran, S. (1984) *Word Processing for Beginners*, Granada Publishing, London.

Diringer, D. (1962) *Writing: Ancient Peoples and Places*, Thames and Hudson, London.

Douglas, J., Reeson, B. and Ryan, M. (1988) Computer microtechnology for a severely disabled preschool child. *Child: Care, Health and Development*, **14** (2) 93–104.

Drage, C. and Evans, N. (1988) Something special. Hardware like the concept keyboard gives special needs kids the chance to use the micro. But what software is there? *Acorn User*, **69**, 27–9.

Drage, C. and Evans, N. (1988) Press for action. Part two of our review of concept keyboard's software for children with special needs. *Acorn User*, **70**, 90–101.

Drage, C. and Evans, N. (1988) Please do touch. More and more pieces of software use Microvitec's Touchscreen to make them easier to use for children, but how good are they? *Acorn User*, **68**, 159–61.

Fairhurst, M.C. and Maynard, C.A., An electronic aid for teaching writing and drawing skills. *Child: Care, Health and Development*, **4** (5) 285–90.

Flewitt, P. (1985) *Word Processing: An Introduction*, 2nd edn, Macmillan, London.

Foster, L. (1988) Writers' workshops, the word processor and the psychiatric patient. *British Journal of Occupational Therapy*, **51** (6) 191–2.

Fraser, K. (1985) *Word Processing and Typing*, Usborne Publishing, London.

Fussey, G. (1983) Teaching typing to children with cerebral palsy. *British Journal of Occupational Therapy*, **46** (11) 321–3.

Gillon, R. and Holloway, I. (1982) A painting easel for the severely handicapped. *British Journal of Occupational Therapy*, **45** (12) 386–7.

Goodnow, J. (1977) *Children's Drawings*, Open Books, London.

Green, G. (1987) Nothing special? Micro computing with children who have physical handicaps. *A & B Computing*, **4** (9) Educational supplement.

Griffiths, I.D. and Craft, A.W. (1988) Management of juvenile chronic arthritis. *Hospital Update*, **14** (4) 1372–84.

Hamilton, A.M. and Shah, S.K. (1984) Physical hand function with spina bifida myelomeningocele. *British Journal of Occupational Therapy*, **47** (5) 147–50.

Hammond, R. (1984) *The Writer and the Word Processor*, Coronet Books, Hodder and Stoughton, London.

Handley, J. (1986) Posture education in primary schools. *Health at School*, **1** (6) 176–7; **1** (7) 220–1; **1** (8) 259–60.

Harpin, P. (1981) *With a Little Help: Volume 4, Household and Seating; Volume 5, Communication*, The Muscular Dystrophy Group of Great Britain, Nattrass House, 35 Macaulay Road, London SW4 0QP.

Hawkridge, D., Vincent, T. and Hales, G. (1983) *New Information Technology in the Education of Disabled Children and Adults*, Croom Helm, London.

Heaton, A. (1987) Primary value of word processing. *Micro User*, **5** (1) 65.

Hope, M.H. (1987) *Micros for Children with Special Needs*, Souvenir Press, London.

Isard, M. (1988) Art comes undone. *Acorn User*, **69**, 98–103.

Jarman, C. (1977) A helping hand for slow learners. *Special Education – Forward Trends*, **4**, 11–13.

Jarman, C. (1977) *The Development of Handwriting Skills: A Resource Book for Teachers*, Basil Blackwell, Oxford.

King, J.C. (1987) Big, bright and beautiful. By using simple triangles and squares, children can build up complex pictures with Kiddie Art. *Acorn User*, **54**, 87–91.

Legat, M. (1986) *Writing for Pleasure and Profit*, Robert Hale, London.

Morrison, A. (1978) Occupational therapy for writing difficulties in spina bifida children with myelomeningocele and hydrocephalus. *British Journal of Occupational Therapy*, **41** (12) 394–8.

Newell, A.F. (1985) Developing appropriate software. *British Journal of Occupational Therapy*, **48** (8) 242–3.

Newman, J. (1982) An approach to improving handwriting by motor and tactile methods. *British Journal of Occupational Therapy*, **45** (5) 245–7.

Nicol, E. (1976) Typing with my left foot. *Special Education – Forward Trends*, **3** (4) 21–3.

Page, S. and MacAuslan, A. (1978) Poor handwriting and the pencil hold of learning disabled children. *British Journal of Occupational Therapy*, **41** (8) 282–3.

Philip & Tacey Ltd (distributor) (1989) *Write Angle: The Desk Top Writing Aid*, Philograph Publications.

Pickard, P. and Alston, J. (1988) *Helping Secondary School Pupils with Handwriting: Current Research, Identification and Assessment, Guidance*, Supplement to the handwriting file, Alston, J., Taylor, J. LDA, Wisbech, Cambs.

Pitt, N. (1975) Typing for the disabled child. *British Journal of Occupational Therapy*, **38** (6) 132–4.

Renn, G. (1976) Initial investigation into the effect of wrist splinting in children with Still's disease. *British Journal of Occupational Therapy*, **39** (1) 9.

Residents of Delph Manor Hostel, Leeds (1986) *To Camp or Not to Camp?* PRU-Printing and Publishing Unit for Continuing Education, Leeds.

Residents of Delph Manor Hostel, Leeds (1986) *Camping on!* PRU-Printing and Publishing Unit for Continuing Education, Leeds.

RICA (1984) *Communication Aids: A guide for people who have difficulty speaking*, Research Institute for Consumer Affairs (RICA)/Communication Aids Centre (Frenchay Hospital, Bristol), 14 Buckingham Street, London WC2N 6DS.

Routledge, L. (1976) Children's drawings. *British Journal of Occupational Therapy*, **39** (9) 219–21.

Rowe, B. (1981) *Type It Yourself*, Penguin, London.

Sassoon, R. (1983) *The Practical Guide to Children's Handwriting*, Thames and Hudson, London.

Sassoon, R. and Briem, G.S.E. (1984) *Teach Yourself Handwriting*, Hodder and Stoughton, London.

Shannon, F. (1987) *Paper Pleasures: From basic skills to creative ideas*, Mitchell Beazley, London.

Smart, S., Mackenzie, L., Richards, D. (1985) The design of viable software for use in occupational therapy. *British Journal of Occupational Therapy*, **48** (10) 296–8.

Smith, P. (1984) Handwriting and spelling. *Gnosis*, **5**, 24–5.

Somers, D. (1987) Brushing up. Is the microbrush graphics system the natural choice for the professional computer artist? *A & B Computing*, **4** (8) 61–6.

Stananought, D. (1987) Keyboarding: a universal approach to basic typewriting skills. *Chambers Commerce Series*, **4** (8) 61–6.

Stoneman, R. (1985) The potential use of the microcomputer with patients suffering from cerebral vascular accident and head injury. *British Journal of Occupational Therapy*, **48** (6) 163–6.

Taylor, J. (1985) The sequence and structure of handwriting competence: points in the mastery of handwriting. *British Journal of Occupational Therapy*, **48** (7) 205–7.

Thomas, D. (1987) In the print 3: in the field of schools' publishing new and updated products are being released all the time. *A & B Computing*, **4** (6) 62–7.

Thomas, D. (1988) Typesetter! Typesetting comes to the classroom with an innovative new program from Sherston. *A & B Computing*, **5** (1) 79–82.

Thomas, D. (1988) Telling Tales. Write your own best seller with Fairy Tales. *A & B Computing*, **5** (4) 56–8.

Touwen, B.C.L. (1972) Laterality and Dominance. *Developmental Medicine and Child Neurology*, **14**, 747–55.

Turnbull, S. (1988) Art in colour. *Micro User*, **6** (11) 154–5.

Vogler, J. (1987) Down to business. It's no problem driving the latest laser printers with your BBC Micro. *A & B Computing*, **4** (9) 74–80.

Vogler, J. (1988) Desk top publishing. *A & B Computing*, **5** (1) 96-102.

Walmsley, W. and Walmsley, E. (1970) *Pitman Commercial Typewriting*, 7th edn. (ed. A.M. Prince), Pitman Publishing, London.

Webster, J.G., Cook, A.M., Tomkins, W.J. and Vanderheiden, G.C. (1984) *Electronic Devices for Rehabilitation*, Chapman and Hall, London.

Wells, G. (1983) *The Craft of Writing Articles*, Allinson and Busby.

Williams, M. (1970) *Brain Damage and the Mind*, Penguin, London.

Appendix A

Glossary of microcomputing terms

ASCII: American Standard Code for Information Exchange. This code assigns a number between 0 and 255 to every letter character, number and symbol. These numbers are understood by all computers.

BASIC: Beginner's All Purpose Symbolic Instruction Code. One of the languages used for programming computers.

Bidirectional printing: The ability of some printers to print left to right and right to left, which is faster than one which prints in one direction only.

Binary: The basic language used by any computer or word processing system. The system is made up of zeros and ones which are combined in groups of eight or sixteen.

Bit: The smallest unit of computer language.

Bold strike: A technique in which the printer strikes several times so that letter characters appear darker.

Byte: Eight binary bits.

Centring: A facility of word processing which will arrange the required text in the centre of a line.

Chip: A silicon memory unit inside the computer.

CPS: Characters per second. Usually refers to printer speed.

Cursor: A marker on the monitor screen which may be moved to where the next screen operation is required.

Daisy wheel: A system of printing in which a wheel with a spoke for each letter, number or symbol spins round until the required symbol is in position. The spoke is then struck and the symbol printed. This method produces high quality print.

Database: A program which stores information which may be sorted or ordered into various categories.

Disk drive: A device which contains a read/write head which picks up the magnetic information from the disk and transmits it to the computer memory or the printer.

Disk operating system (DOS): The main program of a microcomputer or word processor.

Dot matrix printer: A type of printer in which the symbols are printed by means of a number of pins on the printing head. The print is thus formed by a number of dots so the print is not as solid as that formed by a daisy wheel printer. It is a fast method of printing.

Double strike: A printing technique in which characters are printed twice, thus producing bolder more clearly defined text.

Elite: Print with 12 characters to the inch.

Embedded commands: The format of completed text is determined by such commands inserted in the text.

File: A document stored on floppy disk.

Global search: A facility of word processing which enables the user to locate the occurrences of specific words or symbols.

Graphics: Anything displayed on the screen or monitor which is not text.

Hard copy: A printed copy of a document.

Hardware: The physical parts of the computing or word processing system.

Ink jet printing: A printing system in which ink is sprayed through an electrostatic grid. It is a fast and high quality system, but more expensive than daisy wheel or dot matrix printers.

Interface: A device to connect parts of the computer or word processing system.

Justification: The aligning of the margins of a page of print. Justifying the right margin will give the appearance of a printed page rather than a typewritten one which will have a ragged right margin.

Memory: The microcomputer's or word processor's ability to hold information.

Menu: A facility of word processing which presents a number of options to the user.

Modem: A device used in conjunction with a microcomputer which allows information to be sent or received by telephone to and from other microcomputers.

Monitor: Visual display unit (VDU).

Mouse: A small device which is pushed round the work surface which, when connected to the microcomputer, controls the movements of the cursor.

Peripherals: Any equipment which is connected to the microcomputer.

Pica: Print which has 10 characters to the inch.

Platen: Part of the printer. A roller on which the paper rests while characters are being printed on it.

Pitch: The size of the print.

Proportional spacing: Printing which allows symbols to take up space proportional to its width. Proportional spacing will allow three times as much width for a w as for an i.

Program: A list of instructions which has been written in computer language and which the microcomputer uses to perform tasks.

RAM: Random Access Memory. Computer memory which may be read from or written to.

Read/write head: The arm of the disk drive which reads information from the disk or writes information on it.

ROM: Read Only Memory. The memory on chips within the computer which may be read but not written to.

Software: Programs used with a computer or word processing system.

Spell checker: A program which will search through a file and mark incorrect spellings.

Winchester disk drive: A hard disk drive.

Word wrap: The feature of a word processing program which determines the end of one line of text and the beginning of the next without intervention of the user.

Appendix B

Glossary of medical terms

Abduction: Movement away from the mid-line of the body.

Adduction: Movement towards the mid-line of the body.

Apraxia: Inability to perform certain movements because of lack of ability to plan movements prior to their execution.

Arthrogryposis: A condition in which there is rigidity and immobility of some joints accompanied by absence or malformation of muscle round the joints.

Ataxia: Unsteadiness due to lesions of the cerebellum.

Athetosis: Fluctuating muscle tone and impairment of postural control causing involuntary movements

ATNR: Asymmetrical tonic neck reflex. An abnormal reflex in which turning the head to one side increases extensor hypertonus on the side to which the head is turned and flexor hypotonus on the opposite side.

Atrophy: Wasting, particularly of muscle.

Brittle bones: *see* Osteogenesis imperfecta.

Cerebellar lesion: Damage or injury to the cerebellum, the part of the brain which refines coordination of movement. Lesions may result in ataxia, tremor or speech disorders.

Cerebral palsy: A group of disorders in which there is disturbance of movement.

Congenital: Existing at or before birth.

CVA: Cerebrovascular accident. Stroke.

Diplopia: Double vision.

Disability*: Restriction or lack (resulting from an impairment) of the ability to perform an activity in the manner or within the range considered normal for a human being.

Distal: Situated away from the centre of the body.

Dysarthria: Difficulty with articulation resulting from impairment of neuromuscular control.

Dysfunction: Difficulty with or impairment of a physical or mental function.

Dyspraxia: Difficulty with planning movement at a cerebral level.

---

* Definition from Wood, P.H.N. (1980) Appreciating the consequences of disease: the International Classification of Impairments, Disabilities and Handicaps. *WHO Chronicle*, **34**, 376–80.

Dystonia: Disturbance of muscle tone causing uncontrolled writhing movements.

Dystrophy: An actively destructive disorder.

Extension: The movement of stretching out a part of the body.

Fine motor: Relating to precise movement usually of the hands.

Flaccid: Soft and flabby, lacking tone.

Flexion: Bending, the opposite of extension.

Gross motor: Relating to large movements.

Handicap*: A disadvantage for a given individual (resulting from an impairment or disability) that limits or prevents fulfilment of a role that is normal (depending on age, sex and social and cultural factors) for that individual.

Hemianopia: A condition in which only half of the visual field is intact.

Hemiplegia: Paralysis of the limbs on one side of the body due to impairment of the opposite cerebral hemisphere.

Hydrocephalus: An increase in the volume of fluid in the ventricles of the brain due to obstruction of pathways through which it normally drains.

Impairment*: Loss or abnormality of psychological, physiological or anatomical structure or function.

Interphalangeal: Between the phalanges, the bones of the fingers and toes.

In utero: In the womb.

JCA: Juvenile chronic arthritis.

Lateral: Relating to one side.

Lesion: An injury, wound or structural change.

Motor: Movement, usually related to muscles or the enervation of such muscles.

Multiple sclerosis: A degenerative disease of the nervous system, characterized by scattered patches of hardened glial tissue.

Neurological: Pertaining to nerves.

Occupational therapy: The treatment of physical and psychiatric conditions through specific activities in order to help people reach their maximum level of function and independence in all aspects of daily life.

Oscillatory: Moving to and fro between two points.

Osteoarthritis: A disorder in which there is erosion of the joint cartilage.

Osteogenesis imperfecta: A disorder in which there is congenital fragility of bones.

Parkinson's disease: A progressive disease due to degenerative changes in the cerebral ganglia resulting in increasing muscle rigidity.

Perceptual skills: The ability to process information from sensory input.

Peripheral: On the outside, away from the centre.

Phalanges: Bones of the fingers and toes.

Prone: Lying face downwards.

Pronation: Turning the palm of the hand downwards.

Proximal: Nearest to the centre of the body. The opposite of distal.

Radial: Relating to the radius, the bone which lies along the thumb side of the forearm.

Reflex: An automatic or invariable response to a stimulus.

Rheumatoid arthritis: Chronic inflammation of joints.

* See p. 158 for source of definition.

Sensory: Relating to sensation.

Spasm: A sudden, involuntary contraction of muscle.

Spasticity: A type of muscle rigidity.

Spina bifida: Failure of the bones of the spinal column to unite, which is significant when the spinal cord is exposed to the surface. There is usually partial or complete loss of function below the level of the lesion.

Splint: A device supporting or increasing the function of part of the body.

Supination: Turning upwards, usually referring to the hand when the palm is uppermost.

Supine: Lying on the back with the face upward.

Syndactylism: Webbing of the finger or toes.

Tone: The degree of tension in a muscle.

Tremor: Involuntary trembling of voluntary muscles.

Ulnar: Relating to the ulna, the bone on the inner side of the forearm.

Appendix C

Suppliers

Balans seating	Nottingham Rehab Ltd, 17 Ludlow Hill Road, West Bridgford, Nottingham NG2 1BR, UK
	Nottingham Rehab Ltd, Distributors in USA: Access-Ability, 1307 West 22nd Place, Tulsa, Oklahoma 74107, USA
Biocurve pen	Nottingham Rehab Ltd, 17 Ludlow Hill Road, West Bridgford, Nottingham NG2 1BR, UK
	Nottingham Rehab Ltd, Distributors in USA: Access-Ability, 1307 West 22nd Place, Tulsa, Oklahoma 74107, USA
Book stands	Nottingham Rehab Ltd, 17 Ludlow Hill Road, West Bridgford, Nottingham NG2 1BR, UK

Nottingham Rehab Ltd,
Distributors in USA:
Access-Ability,
1307 West 22nd Place,
Tulsa,
Oklahoma 74107, USA

Fred Sammons Inc.,
Box 32, Brookfield,
Illinois 60513, USA

Chair raisers

Nottingham Rehab Ltd,
17 Ludlow Hill Road,
West Bridgford,
Nottingham NG2 1BR,
UK

Nottingham Rehab Ltd,
Distributors in USA:
Access-Ability,
1307 West 22nd Place,
Tulsa,
Oklahoma 74107, USA

Fred Sammons Inc.,
Box 32, Brookfield,
Illinois 60513, USA

Desk top writing aid
(sloping writing surface)

Philip & Tacey Ltd,
North Way,
Andover,
Hants,
UK

Dycem
(non-slip material)

Nottingham Rehab Ltd,
17 Ludlow Hill Road,
West Bridgford,
Nottingham NG2 1BR,
UK

Nottingham Rehab Ltd,
Distributors in USA:
Access-Ability,
1307 West 22nd Place,
Tulsa,
Oklahoma 74107, USA

	Fred Sammons Inc., Box 32, Brookfield, Illinois 60513, USA
Foam rubber tubing	Nottingham Rehab Ltd, 17 Ludlow Hill Road, West Bridgford, Nottingham NG2 1BR, UK
	Nottingham Rehab Ltd, Distributors in USA: Access-Ability, 1307 West 22nd Place, Tulsa, Oklahoma 74107, USA
	Fred Sammons Inc., Box 32, Brookfield, Illinois 60513, USA
Easiwriter (Whole hand grip)	Nottingham Rehab Ltd, 17 Ludlow Hill Road, West Bridgford, Nottingham NG2 1BR, UK
	Nottingham Rehab Ltd, Distributors in USA: Access-Ability, 1307 West 22nd Place, Tulsa, Oklahoma 74107, USA
Hand strap	Nottingham Rehab Ltd, 17 Ludlow Hill Road, West Bridgford, Nottingham NG2 1BR, UK
	Nottingham Rehab Ltd, Distributors in USA: Access-Ability, 1307 West 22nd Place, Tulsa, Oklahoma 74107, USA

Jenx prone angle chair

Jenx Ltd,
74 Hoyland Road,
Sheffield S3 8AB,
UK

Lap desk

Nottingham Rehab Ltd,
17 Ludlow Hill Road,
West Bridgford,
Nottingham NG2 1BR,
UK

Nottingham Rehab Ltd,
Distributors in USA:
Access-Ability,
1307 West 22nd Place,
Tulsa,
Oklahoma 74107, USA

Microscribe

The Foundation for Communication for
the Disabled,
Foundation House,
Church Street West,
Woking,
Surrey GU21 1DJ,
UK

Microwriter

The Foundation for Communication for
the Disabled,
Foundation House,
Church Street West,
Woking,
Surrey GU21 1DJ,
UK

Pencil grips
Triangular
Stetro-dimpled

LDA,
Duke Street,
Wisbech,
Cambs PE13 2AE,
UK

LDA,
Distributors in USA:
Didax,
Centenial Industrial Park,
5 Fourth Street,
Peabody,
Mass. 01960, USA

Ideal School Supply,
11000 South Laverge Avenue,
Oak Lawn, Illinois 60453, USA

Lake Shore,
2695 East Dominguez Street,
PO Box 6261,
Carson,
California 90769, USA

Pencil grips

Taskmaster Ltd,
Morris Road,
Leicester LE2 6BR,
UK

Steady Write pen

Steady Write Limited Inc.,
7940 Canterbury Lane,
Plantation,
Florida 33324, USA

Stencils, clear

Taskmaster Ltd,
Morris Road,
Leicester LE2 6BR,
UK

Index

Accommodation, visual 26
Adhesive putty 86
Amniotic bands 35
Anti-glare screen 130
Apert's syndrome 35
Arm rest for typists 108
Arm support, *see* Chairs
Arthrogryposis 7, 35, 158
  and typewriting 97
Artwork, range of techniques 73–5
  and adults 74–5
  and children 73
  and microcomputers 93–4
Assessment of adults 39–45
  gross movement 44
  hand function 44–5
  nature of disability 40
  previous history 40
  seating 43–4
  visual impairment 45
Assessment of children 23–39
  disabling conditions 24–5
  motor difficulties 30–6
  perceptual difficulties 27–8
  position of child and materials
    36–8
  selection of recording tools 38–9
  sensory deficits 25–6

Balans seating 51
Biocurve pen 69
Body image 2, 27
Brittle bones, *see* Osteogenesis
    imperfecta
Brushes 72
  bristles 72
  T-bar 72, 83
  see also Paint, application of

Callipers and pencil skills 37
Cassette recorder 131

Cerebral palsy 31–3
Cerebro vascular accident 8–9
Chairs 46–55
  arm support 51
  Balans seating 51
  dimensions of 46–7
  height 48
  Jenx Prone Angle 51
  seat, non slip 51
  swivel 54–5
Chair raisers 48–50
  extended legs 48
  footrests 49–50
  plastic 48–9
  wooden 48–9
Chalk 78–9
  and dyspraxia 78–9
Chalkboard 78–9
Charcoal 78
Computer, *see* Microcomputer
Concentration 29
Copying shapes 18–19
Crayons 76–7
  aqua 77
  fabric 77
  face paints 77
  fluorescent 76
  metallic 77
  pastels 76
  pencil 75
  wax 76
  see also Wax crayon techniques
Cursor 139, 155
CVA, *see* Cerebro vascular
    accident

Daisy wheel printer 103, 133–4
Deacon, Joseph 2, 95
Developmental level 36
Diplopia 26
Disability 24, 158

Disability, acquired 7–9
  limb deficiency 8
  limitation of movement 8
  loss of muscle power 8
  pain 8
  tremor 8
Disability, congenital 5–7
  dystonia 7
  hemiplegia 5
  limitation of movement 7
  movement 5
  muscle power 7
  see also Dyspraxia
Disability and keyboard skills 96,
    117–18
Disability, multiple 24
Disability and recording
    skills 38–9, 40, 116–17
Disk
  floppy 131–2
  hard 132
Disk drive 131
Dominance, hand, *see* Hand
    preference
Dot matrix printer 132–3
Double-sided tape 86
Drawing board clips 86
Drawing pins 86
Drawing skills
  of adults 3–4
  development of 18–19
  human figure 19
  of infants 2
  in school 3
Dycem 84–5, 86
Dynamic tripod grip 15
Dyspraxia 7, 78–9, 87–8, 158
Dystonia 7, 33
Dystonia musculorum deformans 33

Easels 57
Easiwriter pen 69–70
Editing with word processor 140–2
  centring 141, 155
  embedded commands 142

line space 141
right justification 140–1
  see also Typewriter,
    electronic, right
    justification
spell checker 141, 156
word wrap 141, 157
Electric sockets, position of 42
Employment
  and handwriting 41
  and keyboard skills 41
Erasers 81–2
Erasers, adapted
  bulldog clip 81
  epoxy compounds 81–2
  novelty 82
  on pencil 82
  thermoplastic 81
Eye/hand coordination, *see*
    Hand/eye coordination

Figure/background discrimination
    28
Finance for equipment 41–2
Fine motor skills 14–15, 36
Fingering exercises 120–2
Finger painting 83
Footrests 49–50
Foot switch 144
Form constancy 28
Function keys 140

Gaiters for typist 111
Goad Picture Method 33, 115–16
Graphics, microcomputer 93–4
Gross motor skills 11–14, 36, 44
  head control 11–12
  righting reactions 12
  trunk stability 12
  wrist position 12–13

Hand dominance, *see* Hand
    preference
Hand/eye coordination 12, 28
Hand grip 57–8

Hand preference 19–20
  undecided 20
Hand skills 14–17, 44
  development of 14–15
  see also Pencil skills
Handwriting skills
  adults 1, 3–4, 39
  children 2
  difficulties 4
    and concentration 29
    and spelling 29
    and microcomputers 95
    in school 3
    speed 98
Head control 11–12
Head stick 109–10
Hearing deficits 21, 25
Heel ball 89
Hemianopia 26
Hemiplegia 5, 7
Hooked hand 13–14

Imitating shapes, *see* Copying shapes
Intellectual level 36
Inverted hand position, *see* Hooked
    hand

JCA, *see* Juvenile chronic arthritis
Jenx Prone Angle Chair 51
Joint deformity and keyboard
    skills 97
Joystick 144
Justification, right 104, 140–1
Juvenile chronic arthritis 35

Keyboard 100, 103, 129
Keyboard, expanded 111–12
Keyboard, mini 112
Keyboard skills, teaching 115–25
  aligning paper 123
  carriage return 122
  exercise cards 120–1
  factors to consider 115
  fingering exercises 120–2
  Goad picture method 115–16

home keys 120
  shift key 122–3
  simplified method 118–23
  typing words 121–2
  see also Disability and keyboard
    skills; Word processing,
    learning to use
Keyboard skills for joint deformity
    97
Keyboard skills for one hand 124
Keyboard skills and severe
    disability 125
Keyguard 106–8
  attaching to keyboard 106–7
  homemade 107–8
  uses 106

Lap desks 56–7
Layout with word processor, *see*
    Editing with word
    processor
Left handedness 13–14
Limb deficiency 8
Limitation of movement 8

Maturation 24–5
Memory 21, 41
  visual 28
Memowriter 145
Microcomputer
  keyboard 129
  switches and ports 129
Microcomputer and artwork 93–4
Microcomputer, choosing
    equipment 126–8
  facilities required 127
Microcomputer and impaired hand
    function 143–5
  foot switch 144
  joystick 144
  pressure pad 144
  reflected beam switch 144
  touch switch 144
  wobble stick 144
Microcomputer and peripherals 128

Microscribe 145
Microwriter 145
Minor motor dysfunction 35–6
Monitor 130
 anti-glare screen 130
 controls 130
 and ocular discomfort 130
 resolution 130
 size 130
Motivation 22, 25
Motor planning *see* Praxis
Mouth stick 70–1
Multiple sclerosis 8
Muscular atrophy 7, 8, 33
Muscular dystrophy 7, 8, 33

Nolan, Christopher 1
Nystagmus 26

Ocular discomfort and monitor 130
Osteogenesis imperfecta 7, 159

Page turners 113
Paint, application of 82–4
 fingers 82–3
 finger stall 83
 foam plastic block 83
 roller 84
 stick, foam-tipped 83
 T-stick, foam-tipped 83
 see also Brushes
Paper
 dimensions 38, 58
 orientation of 58–9
 quality 37, 58
Paper for printer 104, 135
 fan fold 135
 roll 135
 single sheet 135
Paper, securing 38, 85–6
 adhesive putty 86
 double-sided tape 86
 drawing board clips 86
 drawing pins 86
 Dycem 86

 Velcro 86
Parkinson's disease 8
Pen 66–71
 ballpoint 67–8
 barrel 66–7
  diameter of 67
  texture of 66–7
 felt-tipped 79–80
 fibre-tipped 68–9
 fountain 68
 nylon and plastic tipped 69
 weight of 66
Pen, adapted
 Biocurve 69
 Easiwriter 69–70
 Steady Write 70
Pen caps 67–8
 safety of 79–80
Pen, friction of 38, 68–9
Pen holder 70–1
 mouth stick 70–1
 thermoplastic 70
 wire 70
Pencil 60–2
 barrel 62
  diameter 62
  shape 62
 hardness 60–1
 pop-a-pencil 62
 propelling 62
 sharpening 61–2
Pencil crayons 75
Pencil grip 15
 dynamic tripod 15
 radial 15
 ulnar 15
Pencil grips 63–6
 ball 64
 dimpled 63
 foam rubber grips 66
 rubber tubing 63–4
 thermoplastic 63
 triangular 63
Pencil skills, development of 2–3
 see also Drawing skills

Perceptual difficulties 21–2, 27–8
  body image 22, 27
  form constancy 28
  position in space 22, 27
  spatial relationships 22, 27–8
Peripherals, *see* Microcomputer and
    peripherals
Peripheral vision 25
Pluckrose, Henry 92
Portability of equipment 42
Position 36–7, 43–4, 46
  constraints due to injury 37
  and pencil skills 37
  sitting 37
  standing 36–7
  working 43
Position in space 22, 27
  of letters and numerals 22, 27
Potential, developmental 24
Praxis 17–18, 30–1, 45
Pressure pad 144
Printer, electronic 105–6
  advantages 105
  disadvantages 105–6
Printer with microcomputer 132–4
  daisy wheel 133–4
  dot matrix 132–3
  paper for 135
  ribbons for 134
  see also Word processing
Printing 92–3
  finger 92
  household objects 93
  potato 92
  rubber stamps 93

Reflected beam switch 144
Ribbons 102–3, 134
Righting reactions 12
Rubbing 89–92
  bark 89
  brass 89
  cast iron 89
  coins 89, 92
  household objects 89

leaves 89
Rulers, adapted 84–5
  with Dycem, folded strip 84–5
  with Dycem sheet 84
  with Dycem spots 84
  with rubber solution 84

Scanning devices 112
Scott, Guy 83
Seating 43
  custom-made 53
Sensory ability 21
  see also Hearing deficits; Visual
      acuity; Visual defects;
      Visual scanning
Spatial relationships 27
Spatial skills 22, 27–8
Spelling difficulties 29
Splints for typists 111
Sponge rubber tubing 63–4
Stability 30, 43, 46
  see also Hand grips; Position
Standing frames and boxes 53
Stand for book, paper 113–15
Steady Write pen 70
Stencils 86–9
  geometric shapes 87–8
  of objects 88
  uses of 87–8
  waxed card 88
Stroke, *see* Cerebro vascular
    accident
Syndactilism 35

Telephone index 112–13
Templates 88–9
Touch switch 144
Tremor 8, 33
Trolley for microcomputer 57
Trunk stability 12
T-stick 83, 110
Tunnel vision 25–6
Typewriter
  and impairment 96–7
  reasons for using 99

Typewriter, electric 101–2
  advantages 101
  disadvantages 101–2
Typewriter, electronic 102–4
  illuminated display 103–4
  keys 103
  paper feed 104
  power supply 102
  ribbons for 102–3
  right justification 104
  see also Editing, right justification
Typewriter, manual 99–101
  advantages of 100
  disadvantages of 100–1
Typing stick 110–11
  strap for 111
  T-stick 110

V.D.U., *see* Monitor
Velcro 86
Visual acuity 45
Visual deficits 25–6
Visual display unit, *see* Monitor
Visual fields, impairment of 25
Visual scanning 21, 26

Wax crayon techniques 92
  grated 92
  notched 92
  with paint 92
Wedge for keyboard 108–9
Wobble stick 144
Word processing 135–8

advantages of 136
chip 136
dedicated word processors 135
disadvantages of 137–8
disk 136
learning to use 138
types of program 136–7
Word processing, additional
      facilities 138–42
  cursor 139, 155
  function keys 140
  menu facilities 138–9
  review of text 138
  storage and retrieval 138
  see also Editing with word
      processor
Word processing for
      children 142–3
  group work 143
Word processor, portable 145
  Memowriter 145
  Microscribe 145
Working surface 37, 47–8
  angle of 47, 56
  with cut out 54–5
  semi-circular 5
  shape 54
  see also Easels; Lap desks;
      Trolley for microcomputer
Wrist position
  for handwriting 12–13
  for keyboard 12–13
WYSIWYG 139